I Have Parkinson's Disease, but Parkinson's Disease Doesn't Have Me

To: Helga

Thanks for your help

Mark I Johnson

A Memoir By
Mark I. Johnson

First published in 2018

ISBN: 9781729171530

Edited by Sean Donovan – www.Seandon.com

For more information, contact:
Mark I. Johnson
1316 3rd Street
Edgewater, Fl. 32132
386-690-8098
marko_nsb@yahoo.com

Printed in the United States of America

I dedicate this book to my wife Beverly, who did not plan on having to deal with my Parkinson's disease any more than I did. Still, she has stood by me through thick and thin. I love you sweetheart.

Contents

Introduction

This is a tale of Parkinson's disease; not its cause or cure, but how some of its sufferers, like me, face the challenges that come with this chronic neurological disease.

It is not meant to offer medical advice on the various treatment options that are available, although it does delve into deep brain stimulation—nor does it tout itself as the definitive work on the subject. These pages contain a layman's perspective on some of the ways Parkinson's patients can deal with emotional, psychological and physical issues that arise from the disease. It is my hope that, by exploring this topic and sharing my experiences, other sufferers of this neurological disaster, or "Parkies" as I call us, will be inspired to get the most they can out of life. For as one caregiver put it, "things could always be worse."

I equate Parkinson's disease to one of life's curveballs and I consider myself a batter. For me, striking out is not an option. In the more than a decade since my own diagnosis, I have swung at many pitches, missing a few, but I've accomplished some hits as well. I credit most of these successes to the inspiration provided by my fellow Parkinson's sufferers and their caregivers. To these individuals, I want to express my profound gratitude; it is through their examples of perseverance, determination, and spirit that I have found the strength I needed to keep fighting this most personal battle and say, "I have Parkinson's disease, but Parkinson's disease doesn't have me."

Chapter 1:
There Must Be Some Mistake

"You have young-onset Parkinson's disease." I first heard those words more than 12 years ago while sitting in the exam room of a doctor's office in New Smyrna Beach, Florida.

I was there for what I thought was a routine examination for a suspected case of carpal tunnel syndrome. My left hand had developed a weird twitch and there was an unfamiliar hesitancy in my fingers as they flew across my computer keyboard while I reported the news as a 45-year-old journalist for The Daytona Beach News-Journal, a mid-sized newspaper on the east coast of central Florida.

"It is a chronic degenerative neurological disorder, but it is not fatal," Dr. Norberto Martinez Jr., the first of many neurologists I have seen during the past decade, said as he held the plastic model of a dissected human head in his hands. "If you were meant to live until you were 90, you might live to 89 (years old)."

Parkinson's disease is named for the 18th-century British physician James Parkinson (1755-

1824), who first described the symptoms and progression of the disease. It affects the parts of the brain that control voluntary movement. There is an excessive loss of dopamine-producing neurons. This reduction manifests itself through various motor symptoms, the most characteristic of which includes resting tremors of the extremities, bradykinesia (a slowness of movement), postural instability and rigidity. Other symptoms can include gait disturbances and akinesia (the lack of movement, typically of a single body part such as a finger). (The A to Z of Parkinson's Disease by Anthony D. Mosley, M.D., M.S. and Deborah S. Romaine. Copyright 2007, 2008 by Amaranth. Checkmark Books, an imprint of Infobase Publishing. Pages 40, 255, 258-9)

Dr. Martinez went on to explain there is no specific cause for the disorder, just as there is no cure. All doctors can do is treat its symptoms, usually with a cacophony of drugs, each with its own vast array of side effects, like hallucinations and compulsive behaviors.

I was in shock. I thought of Parkinson's as an old person's ailment, not something that affected someone in my stage of life. I still had a wife to support, grandchildren to enjoy, and a career to finish. There must be some mistake.

"Holy crap, are you sure?" I asked.

"Yes, I don't use the P-word lightly," said Dr. Martinez.

Being told I suffered from the celebrity disease du jour (thanks to the likes of former world heavyweight boxing champion, the late Muhammad Ali, former U.S. Attorney General Janet Reno, singer Linda Ronstadt, and actor Michael J. Fox, to name a few well-known Parkinson's victims) which had the potential to steal what remained of my youth and the independence that comes with it, wasn't welcomed news. I had watched as Alzheimer's disease robbed my paternal grandfather of his mind, transforming him from a vibrant senior citizen to a frail bag of bones curled up in his bed. That wasn't something I wanted my grandchildren to experience.

At the urging of my wife, Beverly, and other family members, I sought a second opinion. That neurologist told me he knew I had Parkinson's within five minutes of my walking into his office. He offered me some pills for my symptoms but promised nothing else before ushering me out the door.

Eventually, my sister-in-law, who is also a doctor, suggested I seek the expertise of the physicians and staff at the University of Florida's Center for Movement Disorders and Neurorestoration in Gainesville.

Driving two-and-a-half hours, first north along Interstate 95, then west on State Road 40, a 60-mile, two-lane ribbon of asphalt through the Ocala National Forest, and north again on Interstate 75 to the home of the University of Florida Gators, may not have been convenient, but it did provide the opportunity to be treated by such Parkinson's specialists as Dr. Ramon Rodriguez Cruz, Dr. Michael Okun and neurosurgeon Dr. Kelly Foote, along with the rest of the center's staff. This proved well worth the effort because these individuals not only offered me the latest in treatment options and medications, but also the emotional support I needed. I was scared of what the future might hold for me and my family as I began to travel the long road of uncertainty that is Parkinson's.

At the center, I found an unsurpassed level of trust and honesty. Its specialists not only seemed to know what they were talking about, but they were willing to share that knowledge with their patients. At the same time, they didn't try to hide the limitations of what they could do for me. I became so comfortable with the center's doctors and staff that, for a time, they were the only people from whom I would accept advice when it came to my Parkinson's treatment. I even had the bad manners to tell a Daytona Beach-area neurologist that I would not follow his recommendations because they conflicted with the instructions I received in Gainesville.

But, no matter who I see, no one has been able to answer the question that is in the forefront of my mind: "How do I get rid of this disease?" That is likely because no one knows.

Gainesville

In the beginning, my treatment in Gainesville offered little more than I had been promised in New Smyrna Beach.

Dr. Ramon Rodriguez Cruz, the first neurologist I saw at the Center for Movement Disorders, has since left the University of Florida to become the chief of Neurology Service at the

Orlando Veterans Affairs Medical Center and a professor at the University of Central Florida's College of Medicine. He put me on a traditional regimen of Parkinson's medications. These included dopamine agonists like Requip, Neupro and Mirapex, as well as Carbidopa/Levodopa or Sinemet, to help deal with my tremors, rigidity, and fatigue.

But treatment of my symptoms did not stop there. With his larger-than-life personality and ever-ready smile, Dr. Rodriguez Cruz offered hope for an alternative to just living with Parkinson's. He encouraged me to try non-drug avenues like exercise or deep brain stimulation surgery to alleviate my symptoms, along with suggesting I volunteer for clinical trials of experimental drugs and nutritional supplements; all of which led me to believe that one day there might be a breakthrough toward a cure.

My doctor-patient relationship with Dr. Rodriguez Cruz lasted five years. Then, after performing my first deep brain stimulation procedure with Dr. Kelly Foote in 2011, Dr. Michael Okun took over primary supervision of my case.

Dr. Okun, a small, inquisitive man with curly black hair, who Beverly describes as having "one hell of a brain and bedside manner," renewed my confidence that I am on the right track. Not only is he the medical director of the National Parkinson's Foundation and administrative director of the Center for Movement Disorders in Gainesville, but Dr. Okun is also a New York Times bestselling author on the subject of Parkinson's disease.

He graduated with a bachelor's degree in history from Florida State University before earning his medical degree at the University of Florida in 1996.

Dr. Okun is very easy to talk to and is always ready to answer any questions I might have. But most importantly, he speaks at a medical level I can understand. He and Dr. Foote co-founded the Center for Movement Disorders and Neurorestoration at UF in 2002.

Dr. Foote is a native of Salt Lake City, Utah. He earned his undergraduate degree in materials science engineering from the University of Utah College of Engineering. That was followed by his M.D. from Utah's College of Medicine in 1995. He then completed his neurosurgical residency at the University of Florida. In addition, both he and Dr. Okun studied movement disorders neurology at Emory University in Atlanta.

Dr. Foote also trained in deep brain stimulation (DBS) surgery at the Université Joseph Fourier in Grenoble, France, making him one of the few neurosurgeons in the world with fellowship training from both universities. He has performed more than 1,000 DBS surgeries, according to the Center for Movement Disorders' website.

One Hell of a Repair Bill

I suspect my journey with Parkinson's disease began at least two years before I was diagnosed.

Initial hints came as off-the-cuff remarks from friends and acquaintances. "Are you in pain? Did you hurt your back? You seem stiff," they would say to me.

What others saw I could not; a stillness in one arm while walking and/or a slowness getting out of an automobile or rising from a chair. Even as these indicators appeared, I refused to acknowledge them, treating my body in much the same way I do my car—ignoring a problem until something breaks and then expressing shock at the repair bill.

In the beginning, my Parkinson's seemed more of an illusion than a reality to me. I didn't understand what my doctors meant when they spoke of on and off medication cycles or used terms like "postural rigidity." Physically, I felt no different than before my diagnosis. Other than having to remember to take my pills on time, I didn't really think about it much.

Nobody at work cut me any slack because I had a life-altering affliction. I still chased emergency calls that came across the newsroom's police scanner and experienced the bureaucratic boredom that is covering municipal government meetings. And just as I continued to report the news on a daily basis, I was also expected to keep up with my chores at home. The pets needed feeding, the yard needed mowing, dinner needed cooking, and the trash needed to be taken to the curb.

The longer I deal with Parkinson's, the more aware I become of its effects on me—the hesitant steps, the uncontrolled muscle movements, and a difficulty in maintaining my balance. I find I have trouble walking in a straight line, which leads me to ponder what it would be like having to explain to a police officer (who hypothetically pulled me over for suspected drunken driving) that I didn't consume too much bourbon, rather I suffer from a degenerative neurological disorder.

Before being told I had Parkinson's, when I saw someone who jerked as they walked or couldn't keep from spilling a drink due to the tremors in their hands, I would wonder, "What is their problem?" Then I would avert my eyes in an effort to not to let them catch me staring. I would also avoid physical contact as if I was afraid whatever malady they might have was contagious.

Parkinson's changed that. As I became the person who trembled and walked funny, I wanted to hide away so people wouldn't think I was weird. That was until my wife Beverly and I attended a young-onset Parkinson's conference in Atlanta in 2008. There I discovered a whole community of trembling 20 to 60-somethings.

I was so overwhelmed by my fellow "movers and shakers" that I had to turn off my emotional self and revert to my professional self: "Mark I. Johnson, reporter."

Walking among and talking with these individuals, some who moved like they were walking through molasses and others whose extremities jerked like they were swatting mosquitoes in a Florida swamp, it began to dawn on me that I wasn't weird at all. These were people just like me, including a photographer from New York, who was a fellow University of Oregon graduate. They were writers and lawyers, mechanics and merchants.

It was at that moment, despite being terrified I might one day suffer a similar fate, I began to look at my fellow Parkies not out of pity or self-loathing, but with a respect for how these Parkinson's sufferers and their caregivers had learned to deal with this affliction.

One example was a caregiver named Pam, whose husband, Bill, had been twisted into a human pretzel by six years of Parkinson's.

"Parkinson's is an ugly disease," she said.

Yet the couple still attended conferences rather than shutting themselves away from the world. (Daytona Beach News-Journal)

As the years have passed, my symptoms have escalated. The tremor in my left hand grew to a martini-mixing-like shake that encompassed the entire left side my body. A tremor also took root in my right arm, causing my already bad handwriting to become illegible even to me. In addition, the fatigue that is one of Parkinson's most universal symptoms overtook me. By the end of a workday, fingers that once raced across my keyboard, moved like sailors stumbling back to their ship after a shore leave. I would stagger out of the newsroom, physically and mentally exhausted.

I was broken, and despite my attempts to dismiss the signs, I had no choice but to accept the reality that is Parkinson's. Still, witnessing the examples provided by my fellow Parkies has proven to me that our shared disorder affects a person's life, but it does not define it.

Chapter 2:
From the Start

This story begins on a cold January day in Columbus, Ohio, circa 1961.

My parents, Rody and Kathy Johnson, were expecting their second child. Anticipating a daughter, I am told they had decided to name the baby after my mother's mother, Margaret Ingalls Thompson. But when I popped out with all my male parts clearly visible, Margaret Ingalls Johnson quickly became Mark Ingalls Johnson.

Dad had just completed his MBA at the University of Virginia and was embarking on a career in electrical engineering with a Columbus electronics firm. Mom was a stay-at-home mother/artist who had her hands full watching my elder brother by 16 months, Buck, and me.

My parents had met a few years earlier while Kathy was pursuing her undergraduate fine arts degree at the University of Arizona, and First Lt. Rody Johnson was serving out his U.S. Army ROTC commitment at Fort Huachuca, also in Arizona.

I was a challenge from the start, entering the world with cranial stenosis. This is a condition where the bones in an infant's skull fuse together, allowing no space for the brain to grow. Luckily, my doctors were able to remove the offending bits of bone and, other than having a slightly larger than normal head, I suffered no apparent ill effects from the procedure; although I do wonder whether my cranial stenosis played any role in my having Parkinson's. I have no medical evidence of this, but it is something I am curious about. I also ponder whether the pesticides I was likely exposed to while playing in the citrus groves that surrounded my boyhood home, a few years later, may have had a similar effect. Pesticide exposure is another suspected factor in causing Parkinson's disease.

My youthful health issues didn't end with cranial stenosis. I also required surgery to repair a hernia, and twice had my tonsils taken out before celebrating my 10th birthday.

Shortly after the surgery on my skull, Dad's job in Columbus ended. So, he and mom decided to move our little family west to join the aerospace industry boom in southern California.

This was a bit of a homecoming for my mother. She had grown up in Orange County, near Los Angeles, and her parents, C.O. and Margaret Thompson, along with her younger brother Michael, lived there. But, shortly after the birth of my sister Katharine Avis, or Kit, about two years later, the rat race that was southern California became too much for my parents to deal with and they decided to relocate again, this time heading to Florida where my father had been raised.

Dad's parents, Clarence and Florence (better known as Kit and Sis) Johnson, along with a young Rody, had moved in the mid-1930s from Charleston, West Virginia, to the small coastal community of Vero Beach, about an hour north by car from Palm Beach on Florida's east coast. Ulcers had forced my grandfather to leave his family's business, which supplied electrical parts to West Virginia coal mines.

Three decades later, my parents settled our family of five into a single-story, ranch-style home they had built under some majestic live oak trees on two-and-a-half acres of property given to them by my grandfather Johnson (Gramps) in the subdivision he developed around a lake dug from a muck pit a few miles west of town. Kanawha Acres was named for the Kanawha River that flows through Charleston, WV.

Vero Beach

In the early 1960s, Vero Beach, Vero for short, was the kind of town where everybody knew one another. Neighbors were on a first-name basis, and walking into most stores was like visiting an old friend rather than the big-box mentality that prevails today.

It was a great place to grow up as a kid. In addition to running barefoot through the citrus groves that surrounded my neighborhood and fishing for bream or bass in our backyard lake, I could get on my bicycle and pedal from one side of town to the other to visit my grandparents at their home just blocks from the Atlantic Ocean. Sometimes I would stop along the way at the McClure's Drug Store soda fountain downtown for a chocolate malt and egg-salad sandwich.

During these visits, I would often ride in Gramp's golf cart as he cruised the fairways of the Riomar Country Club, swatting little white balls with a 9-iron or fly-fishing for tarpon in the golf course irrigation ponds/water hazards.

I held my first real job in Vero Beach working as a dockhand, lifeguard and grill cook at the Riomar Bay Yacht Club, to which our family belonged. It was also where my dreams of athletic glory went unfulfilled in the city recreation department's youth football and baseball leagues. I didn't fare much better as a member of the Vero Beach High School Fighting Indians football or swim teams either.

Vero was where I pulled the lifeless body of a little boy from a backyard swimming pool during a walk home from the middle school bus stop. On a more positive note, I also kissed my first girl there. It was in Vero Beach where I learned to saltwater fish with my father in the waters of the Indian River Lagoon and the Tarpon Hole. I watched many a Los Angeles Dodgers spring training exhibition game from the left outfield berm under a royal blue, early-spring sky at Dodgertown.

I experienced the civil rights movement in this small, southern town and I joined the "hippie revolution" in a white VW microbus my mother decorated with multi-colored, stick-on flower decals.

As the 1960s turned into the 1970s, Vero Beach and I both grew, as did the Johnson household. To hear Mom and Dad tell that story is quite amusing. They got into a "honeymoon mood" one evening after a cousin's wedding, and nine months later, my younger brother popped out. They used to say that none of their children were planned, but Charlie was the biggest surprise. As Mom was being wheeled into the Indian River Memorial Hospital delivery room, she realized the date was April 1 and could be heard crying out, "I can't do this to one of my children."

According to my parents, Charlie, who is 10 years my junior, was raised by committee. Everyone in the family contributed to his upbringing, including his two older brothers and the stash of Playboy magazines hidden under the mattresses in the bedroom we shared.

From the time he was a toddler, Charlie followed us into the groves. We fished with him in the lake and took him to see one of his first movies. It was at the Florida Theater in downtown Vero Beach, during a showing of the

"Three Musketeers", when a well-endowed actress appeared on the screen, Charlie announced to the audience, "She's got big boobies!"

About this same time, newly constructed homes began sprouting up like weeds adjacent to our neighborhood amid Waldo Sexton's citrus groves and in the cow pastures of John Tripson's dairy farm. Walmart opened the first big box store in Vero Beach and a multitude of new residents descended on this quaint beachside town like a swarm of locusts; bringing with them an attitude of "it's not who you are that matters, but what you have."

A Change of Coasts

As I was about to enter my junior year at Vero Beach High School, Dad was offered the opportunity to transfer back to the West Coast, this time to northern California, and manage a project for Harris Corporation, the aerospace/communications company for whom he worked. So, he packed the six of us into the family's Mercury Monarch and we headed to Palo Alto in the San Francisco Bay area, with stops along the way in New Orleans and at the Grand Canyon.

Going from Vero Beach High School to Palo Alto High School, "Paly" for short, was like going from kindergarten to college. It was located across the street from Stanford University and some of that esteemed institution's reputation for high academic standards had rubbed off on the lower school.

Paly was where this skinny, weird, Florida kid transformed into the geek with a camera. For the first time in my life, I seemed to fit in.

As Dad's project wrapped up and he prepared to take our clan back to Vero Beach in fall of 1978, I decided I didn't want to go. I had found a place where I belonged, so I talked my parents into letting me stay in California to complete my senior year at Paly. This was made possible because I was taken in by Jennifer Stephens, the high school's dean of students' secretary. She was a wonderful woman who had a warm spot in her heart for a wayward spirit as she welcomed me into her extended family.

Upon graduating from high school in the spring of 1979, with the "Rachel P. Austin Most Improved English Student" award, I departed

Palo Alto and headed to the "Berkeley of the Northwest", Eugene, Oregon, where I became a University of Oregon Duck.

During the next four years, in between playing rugby for the university's club team and photographing everything in sight, I cemented the building blocks of my future career working as a photographer for the UO sports information department and yearbook; while at the same time earning a Bachelor of Science degree in journalism.

Diversity was the backbone of my studies at Oregon's School of Journalism, for it required a broad spectrum of classes, only a third of which could directly focus on my major. So, being my mother's son, I decided to try my hand in the arts. The cocky, wanna-be photojournalist that I was, I told my fine art photography instructor, Willie Osterman, that I wanted to learn "that art stuff."

Luckily for me, this protégé of Ansel Adams indulged my ego and took up the challenge. Willie not only opened my eyes to a different way of seeing the world, but he taught me the techniques needed to translate that vision into an image on film. This helped me understand that a photograph could capture more than an event or a moment in history, but it is also able to stand alone as a piece of art.

In addition to the arts, I studied science, math, history and psychology. I even took a course in wilderness safety and ethics, which I failed because I couldn't get the hang of reading topographical maps. Despite lacking those three credits, which I made up a few months later by taking a Spanish class at a community college, I graduated with my class in the of spring 1983, and stepped into the uninviting job market of a timber depression in the Great Northwest.

Finding no employment opportunities there, I packed my silver Honda Civic sedan until it overflowed, and began the long cross-country drive east, stopping at numerous newspapers along the way, looking for a position as a photojournalist.

Back East

After driving diagonally across the United States, the only job opening I found was at a small, weekly newspaper on Sanibel and Captiva islands, a Southwest Florida resort community where my family had vacationed for years.

I had gone there to visit my grandparents at Shell Point Village, the Fort Myers-based assisted-living facility where they had moved so Nana could get help dealing with Gramps' Alzheimer's disease.

As staff photographer for "The Islander," I quickly earned a reputation of "being everywhere on the islands there was news and lots of places there wasn't." I also began to develop my skills as a reporter, writing stories to accompany my photographs.

Eventually, I came to the conclusion that a person can take only so much sunshine and tropical breezes. Two years after my arrival, I left Sanibel to spend a couple of weeks backpacking through Europe with my older brother Buck who, in 1985, was a U.S Army lieutenant stationed in Germany.

This was followed by a handful of jobs, some successful and others not so much. Then, in 1987, I settled in New Smyrna Beach, Florida, where I had been hired as the staff photographer, late-night sports desk editor, arts & entertainment editor, and jack-of-all-trades for an award-winning, five-day-a-week community newspaper. During the next dozen or so years, I worked my way up to the position of associate editor of "The Observer."

Family

While I was settling into a career, my personal life also solidified with my marriage to Beverly Ann Kinney. I met this native daughter of Maryland while sticking my nose where it didn't belong into her city hall office in Edgewater, a town just south of New Smyrna Beach.

Wandering the halls of the city administration building in search of a story one day, I noticed pictures of a cute blonde accompanied by two boys hanging on a wall in the planning department. At first, I dismissed the blonde as married because of the kids. But after a little investigating, I discovered the woman in the photographs, was not only single, but also available, so I asked Beverly out on a date.

A year passed with our courtship having its ups and downs. At one point, I broke things off to see if something would develop with a former girlfriend. When that foolishness ended, I came crawling on my knees, begging Beverly to take me back.

A few more months of dating passed, then Beverly added a wrinkle of her own to our pairing when she announced her younger son, Brian, wanted to come live with her. Beverly is seven years my senior and had been previously married. Brian was living with his father in Maryland at the time.

Beverly was initially worried Brian would become too attached to me, so we slowed our relationship down for a time, but eventually the three of us moved into a 1920s-era, two-story wooden house near downtown New Smyrna Beach. There we lived as a family for almost a year. Just as I was about to ask for her hand in marriage, Beverly beat me to the punch when she said to me, "What would you say if I said I wanted to get married?

So, I asked her to become my wife.

Upon learning I had proposed to his mother, Brian, who by then was a prepubescent seventh-grader at New Smyrna Beach Middle School, immediately inquired what he would have to call me. While living with his father, Brian had been required to address his stepmother as "Mom," something he despised. So, he wanted to know if I wanted him to address me as "Dad."

Knowing how he felt about the idea, I responded with, "You can call me anything, but ass%#@*."

Brian is not the only family member Beverly brought to our coupling. She also has an older son, Rob, who lived in Maryland with his father and stepmother until he graduated high school and joined the U.S. Navy, where he was a plank holder on the destroyer USS Stout. And then there is her mother, Anna Butts.

Anna is the reason we settled in Central Florida. Beverly had made it abundantly clear from the beginning of our relationship that she would not leave the area as long as her mother was alive. So, with some financial help from Anna and my "Nana" Johnson, Bev and I bought a house in Edgewater.

As the years progressed, so did my relationship with Bev's boys. Rob, who made me a grandfather at the tender age of 39 when he married a local woman and adopted her daughter, began calling me "Pop." Brian and I really bonded as well.

Eventually, I announced to the world in my newspaper column that I was unofficially adopting the boys as my own. As usual, I was a little behind the curve. When I showed the article to Brian and Rob, their reaction was, "What took you so long? We adopted you years ago."

The Reporter in Me

While this was taking place, I matured professionally too. The photojournalist in me slowly evolved away from the camera into more of a straight reporter/editor role. This meant I moved up the career ladder; until, in 1999, my boss at "The Observer," Jim Jones, encouraged me to jump ship.

"It is time for Mark to leave the nest," Jim said during one of my last performance reviews.

I applied and was hired for an opening in the Southeast Volusia bureau of the area's primary newspaper, the Daytona Beach News-Journal. For the next seven years, first in its New Smyrna Beach office, rising to the position of assistant bureau chief, then as a senior reporter in the News-Journal's main Daytona Beach newsroom, I cultivated a reputation as the "Robo-Reporter," covering law enforcement and municipal government. I wrote stories that ranged from personality profiles of local celebrities, to tales of murder and mayhem, to the happenings at municipal planning and zoning board meetings—all of this in addition to writing a weekly column.

Everything seemed to be percolating along smoothly until, in the fall of 2006, I heard the words that would forever change my life; "You have Parkinson's disease."

Chapter 3:
Play the Cards You are Dealt

One of the keys to living with Parkinson's is learning to accept the cards fate has dealt you; while at the same time, not giving in to what Michael J. Fox calls a "neurological catastrophe." I found I could do this by using the skills acquired during more than 30 years in journalism to channel how I felt about my Parkinson's into a book. And I am not alone in seeking such an outlet, according to Hardy Jones and Doug Vanderlaan, motivational speakers I heard during a Parkinson's disease conference in 2016.

Both men were successful in their respective careers prior to being diagnosed with Parkinson's. Jones, as a filmmaker, focused on dolphins, whales and the world's oceans. And Vanderlaan, as a scientist, developed contact lenses with more than 60 US. patents to his credit. It is how these two men handled the news of their illnesses that caught my attention.

They were determined not to give in to this debilitating illness.

Jones, a tall, rail-thin man, said his outlet came with the discovery of a love for painting during a trip to France about a year after his 2012 diagnosis. He said he and his wife were visiting a region along the Seine River that was home to and the inspiration for many of the famous Impressionist painters, when he decided to take a watercolor class.

"I finished a painting in that class and took it back to my wife," the 73-year-old recalled. "She said it wasn't all that bad... I felt like a kid coming home from school with something to put on the refrigerator door."

Upon returning to his St. Augustine Beach, Florida home, Jones continued to paint. That led to another art class and more positive responses. He was hooked.

Today, Jones paints with acrylics, doing still-lifes, landscapes and portraits. He attributes this newfound creativity to the dopamine found in the medication used to treat his Parkinson's symptoms.

"Dopamine lowers inhibitions and enhances artistic tendencies," he said.

However, Jones warned how that same dopamine can also lead to a loss of impulse control like kleptomania, compulsive gambling and/or hyper-sexuality.

"I am delighted (mine) led to painting," he quipped.

Painting also helped Jones overcome the apathy he sometimes feels as a result of his Parkinson's. He said he will get "a spark of inspiration" from something as simple as mixing two colors of paint together to achieve the desired hue. The next thing he knows, he has been at his easel for a couple of hours.

"The experience of painting (also) quiets my tremors and lifts my mood," he said.

As Jones presented some of his artwork, he mentioned another adaptation he has mastered—training himself to paint with his left hand when the Parkinson's tremor in his right wrist bothers him.

"And I am not a lefty," Jones said.

Vanderlaan didn't find a new outlet after his diagnosis; instead, Parkinson's led him to channel a 40-year love affair with music in a new direction—raising people's awareness about the disease.

He and his musical partner joined Team Fox, an affiliate of the Michael J. Fox Foundation, to hold a fundraiser for Parkinson's research. He said participants bid to have the duo sing a favorite tune, and a "lot more" ($100 minimum, if the pair had to learn the requested song from scratch).

The Michigan native, who looks more scientist than songster, said his interest in music began as a youngster. According to Vanderlaan, growing up he idolized his 17-year-old brother, who had a guitar and record player.

"He was very, very cool to an 11-year-old," the scientist said.

As one might expect, the elder Vanderlaan told his younger brother, "in no uncertain terms," to stay out of his room and leave the guitar alone. But, since his older sibling was not home most of the time, Vanderlaan said he would frequently sneak in to play the instrument and use his records. When the elder sibling finally caught on and realized his little brother could properly care for the items, he decided to allow him to use them. Eventually, he sold the guitar to his younger brother.

"It was a terrible guitar," Vanderlaan quipped. But he used it to learn a few basic chords, then some songs, and that led to his life-long love affair with music and singing.

Over the years, the Jacksonville, Florida resident said he formed musical groups with friends and learned to play other instruments, which led to performances in churches and, eventually, neighborhood coffee houses.

Ironically, it was through the guitar that Vanderlaan learned of his illness.

"I was practicing in my home and my right hand developed a mind of its own (during a particularly spirited guitar riff)," he said. When he got the tremor in his right wrist checked, it was confirmed as Parkinson's. That was eighteen months ago.

"I knew about Parkinson's because I had two uncles with it," he said

Despite his diagnosis, Vanderlaan remains determined to make music. He said whenever his Parkinson's interferes with his playing, he contacts his neurologist for advice on how to deal with the symptoms.

"He tells him to keep on strumming," he said.

Vanderlaan knows the day will come when he will no longer be able to play the guitar, but he vows to use other methods, such as a computer, to make music. He isn't going to let Parkinson's silence him, even if he has to resort to brain surgery.

"Music gives me a reason to keep pushing back against my Parkinson's," Vanderlaan said.

Chapter 4:
Look, No Tremors

I first learned about Deep Brain Stimulation from a family friend, attorney Larry Barkett, while visiting my parents in Vero Beach. He also suffers from Parkinson's disease.

Deep Brain Stimulation (DBS) is a therapy involving surgical implantation of electrodes into specific areas of the brain that are responsible for movement. This allows for transmission of an electrical current into these areas. The current stimulates these, reducing symptoms such as tremors and rigidity. (The A to Z of Parkinson's Disease. pages 80-81. Anthony D. Moseley, M.D., M.S. and Deborah S. Romaine. 2007 Checkmark Books).

Upon hearing I had been diagnosed with Parkinson's, Larry made the effort to approach me outside my parents' church after Sunday services. He explained how his life had changed since undergoing the DBS procedure.

"Look, no tremors," he said holding out his hands by way of a greeting.

Here was a man who had confronted his affliction and done something about it. This gave me pause from automatically dismissing the idea that some good might come from having someone stick things into my brain. Still, it is was a long way from a strange twitching of my left hand to hearing I might need brain surgery.

Larry didn't sugar-coat his description of the procedure. He spoke of being awake during the surgery, during which four electrodes at the end of a hair-thin wire, or lead, are inserted into a specific area of the brain through a hole a surgeon drills in the patient's skull. He explained that being awake is necessary, so the surgeon can communicate with the patient and know he is implanting the lead in exactly the right spot. These electrodes emit a minute electrical current that compensates for the loss of dopamine-producing neurons in the brain caused by Parkinson's disease. Dopamine helps control voluntary muscle movement.

While the National Parkinson's Foundation acknowledges it is not fully known why deep brain stimulation works, research has shown its benefits; primarily the reduction or elimination of Parkinson's motor symptoms, such as tremors. Results can last more than 10 years.

In addition to talking about DBS positives, Larry also spoke about possible side effects caused by the surgery. His speech became so garbled he had to give up litigating in court because people could no longer understand him. Still, he talked about the therapy in such positive terms, saying the treatment had given him back some semblance of a normal life.

Based on this information, and after consulting with my own movement disorder specialist, Beverly and I decided to proceed with the first of my two Deep Brain Stimulation surgeries at Shands Hospital at the University of Florida in 2011, five years after my initial Parkinson's diagnosis.

The most painful part of the procedure was when a halo-like, metal frame was screwed onto my skull. This is used to keep a patient's head still during the surgery, thus allowing for precise placement of the electrodes into the brain.

That's not all I felt during the four-plus-hour operation, however. There was also a sensation when the surgeon cut into my scalp and scraped a pocket of flesh away from the bone to make room for the wire connected to the electrodes he implanted in the subthalamic nucleus on the right side of my brain. I also heard and felt pressure from the drill bit as it bore through my skull; it sounded like the neurosurgeon was drilling into concrete.

Being conscious during the operation led to unexpected discomforts as well.

As I was being wheeled into the operating room on a gurney, a member of the surgical team asked me what type of music I would like to listen to during the procedure. "Classic rock," I replied. That is when I was informed this was also my neurosurgeon, Dr. Kelly Foote's, musical choice. Little did I know the irony of my selection.

Just as Dr, Foote began to drill into my skull, Don McLean's rock anthem "American Pie" flowed through the surgical suite sound system. When McLean sang the line, "and this will be the day that I die," I lost all semblance of composure and reverted into a blubbering mass of tears.

"Beverly," I cried out, thinking I might never see my wife again.

I told the hospital's staff of this musical misfortune prior to my second DBS surgery a couple of years later. Ironically, a song by the artist that inspired "American Pie" with a similar lyric; Buddy Holly's "That'll Be the Day", flowed from the operating room speakers. This time, however, nurses went scurrying for the mute button, much to my amusement.

It is hard to describe what thoughts ran through my mind when the neurologist began experimenting with the various power settings and frequencies of electrical current being fed into the electrodes implanted in my brain in an effort to quiet my tremor. As tingling sensations coursed down my arm, he asked whether I was able to control my twitching left hand. One moment it jerked incessantly, then suddenly it laid still on the stainless-steel table-top, responding to the orders given to it by my brain.

Once the correct power setting was programmed into the pulse-generator implanted in the right-side of my chest like a pacemaker, the hole in my skull was plugged and off to the recovery room I went. A month or so later, I returned to the hospital to be wired up to the battery-powered generator in my chest. This provides the electric current for the electrodes.

In 2013, I had the procedure repeated on the left side of my brain, calming the tremor on the right side of my body. This time I knew what to expect, and the surgery went smoother (with the exception of the musical snafu).

I was so relaxed during that operation that I was tempted to ask the resident sitting in a back corner of the operating room reading a book, to turn to its last page and let me know how the operation would turn out. I did have the presence of mind to warn the two student observers in the operating theater, "this is what happens if you are bad," as the neurosurgeon began to drill into my skull. (Daytona Beach News-Journal)

Like Larry's, my surgeries have not been without side effects. My voice has become muffled. I also suffer from the loss of some cognitive function such as memory. I also have problems with my balance, but these were risks I knew and accepted going in.

In the years since my 2013 surgery, as I traveled to Gainesville to have my second pulse generator fine-tuned, I also began noticing new

Parkinson's symptoms I had never noticed before, such as the on and off of my medications, when Parkinson's drugs are at their most effective (on) and least effective (off). My gait, too, has become more hesitant when it comes time to take my carbidopa/levodopa, which I do every three hours throughout the day. And what I believe is dyskinesia, or involuntary muscle movements, has appeared in my left arm when I exercise. I also have tremors in my left leg; leading to the sensation, at times, that I am tap dancing while sitting still.

I don't know if my experiences are typical; although in talking with other Deep Brain Stimulation recipients, I have discovered their results, like Parkinson's disease symptoms, can vary greatly from patient to patient.

One such individual is Marilyn, a South Florida-based freelance journalist. When she considered Deep Brain Stimulation therapy, or "filling her head with wires" as she likes to call it, Marilyn said she believed DBS would give her back a little of the life Parkinson's had stolen from her. But first, Marilyn had to do something she had never done before; let go of control.

"Brain surgery... was not on my bucket list," Marilyn wrote in a 2015 Washington Post newspaper article about her fight with Parkinson's.

When she showed positive results from the surgery, the elimination of her tremors and dystonia, it gave her a new outlook on life. Dystonia is an involuntary muscle contraction that causes contorted limbs or abnormal postures.

"Denial, anger and bargaining were replaced by relief, amazement and disbelief," Marilyn wrote. (Washington Post, 2015)

Not everyone's outcome was as positive.

More than 20 years of Parkinson's had left Gisela (she asked her last name not be used) with muscle tremors on the left side of her body and robbed the Port Orange, Florida resident of much of her balance. When medication no longer helped with the problems, she underwent Deep Brain Stimulation surgery in 2008.

"I figured it couldn't hurt," she said. (Daytona Beach News-Journal, 2011)

While the surgery quieted the tremors, it did little, if anything, for her balance. As a result,

Gisela said if she had the chance to do it over again, she might not.

Still, other recipients have faced even bigger challenges.

Chapter 5:
There are No Promises

When talking about his history with Parkinson's disease, John Mirabella speaks in a soft, steady voice, although his body is anything but still while seated in the straight-backed chair on which his 6-foot, 3-inch tall frame rests. Parkinson's has the 60-plus-year-old Port Orange resident squirming and jerking. First, he crosses one leg, then the other, and his hands are in constant motion.

I met John and his wife, Pat, while attending a "Dance for PD" exercise class at a local YMCA. Being closer to my age than the rest of the class's participants, and due to the fact John had also undergone Deep Brain Stimulation surgery, I wanted to know more about his battle with Parkinson's. So, we sat down, and he told me his story.

John first became aware of his affliction at the age of 52 when Pat noticed his left arm hung motionless when he walked.

"It didn't swing anymore," he said of this typical Parkinson's symptom.

There were earlier indications as well, like trouble with his bowels. John said he suffered from constipation and the associated hemorrhoid problems for some time prior to being diagnosed.

"My doctor said your Parkinson's (likely) started in your intestines," the father of two recalled. Although in the beginning, he said this did not bother him too much. "My intestines were always on the lazy side."

It was the way the couple received the news of John's illness, they said, that was the most troubling part of the diagnosis.

Rather than sitting down and explaining his illness to him, John said his doctor just walked up to him and announced, "You have Parkinson's disease and there isn't much you can do about it."

Things weren't much different for Pat, John recalled.

"My doctor came out of the (examination) room and told her, "Your husband has Parkinson's'."

"I wanted to wring his neck," Pat, a former nurse, said.

At first, John did not realize how severe a problem he faced.

"I didn't really understand Parkinson's. Sometimes you hear things and they just fly right over your head. I had to have Pat explain to me what it was," he said.

Looking back on the past dozen or more years with this disorder, Pat, with the help of a journal she has kept since 2002, now recognizes the many stages of the disease John has gone through.

"It is amazing," Pat said of the information contained in her four-by-six-inch notebook. "I started listing everything," including when John told his friends and children about his illness and his visits to the emergency room. She even wrote of the mornings when her husband couldn't walk into the living room of their home.

"He would crawl," she said. "I didn't want to see him (that way)."

Despite "taking them like candy," John said he didn't respond well to the medications he was prescribed for his symptoms. He consumed as many as 16 pills a day until the couple decided to seek an alternative means of dealing with his Parkinson's. That is when they discovered Deep Brain Stimulation (DBS) therapy.

The couple said they learned about the procedure through stories in the newspaper and on television, as well as doing research on the internet. Since John's general health appeared to make him a good candidate for the procedure, they broached the subject with his neurologist, who agreed to look into it.

"He said it should help me, but there were no promises," said John.

He said his doctor decided to implant one lead into his brain, affecting only the left side of John's body, then judge that outcome before proceeding with a second lead.

While surgery did address some symptoms, halting the dragging and slapping of John's left foot when he walked, it was not without its problems. Pat said John had a stroke, a bleed in the brain, during the operation. This is a noted risk factor with DBS surgery.

"What was supposed to be a four-hour surgery took like seven hours," she said. "I was freaking out."

After the operation, John was placed in the hospital's intensive care unit where he didn't know Pat's or his own name. She said he called her "Loretta" and couldn't tell her the time of day.

"He was like a baby for me to take care of," Pat said. "The first time he called me by my name, I cried."

In addition to the stroke, Pat said John developed a fever while in the ICU, which meant more time in the hospital undergoing a series of antibiotic treatments.

Medical issues aside, John has faced other challenges due to Parkinson's, including how to financially support his family.

"I was a carpenter," John said of his pre-Parkinson's occupation. "I liked building things and doing things with my hands."

The former Long Island, N.Y., resident said he continued to work for about a year after his diagnosis, but when John began getting injured on the job, a co-worker pointed out he may be eligible to receive government disability. It took two years for that paperwork to come through, he said.

For a time, John kept busy doing projects around his house or for friends, but eventually those jobs became less and less common.

"I look at my tools and I don't even want to touch them," he now says.

And that is not all that has changed.

"We used to go camping a lot," John said of a former favorite family activity. "I miss doing those things. Now that I have Parkinson's, I am not as free anymore."

But he doesn't just sit around the house. John lends a hand with household chores by keeping up with the laundry and vacuuming.

"I would rather be doing something than just staring at the walls. That gets boring after a while," he quipped. And despite depending on a cane to maintain his balance, John also has to deal with the sudden freezing of his feet when they refuse to move while walking, sometimes abruptly in mid-step; yet another symptom of Parkinson's. John said he stays physically active by participating in "Dance for PD" classes with Pat twice a week and goes to the gym with neighbors three times a week.

John is not alone in being affected by Parkinson's; life has changed for Pat as well. According to her, the couple used to come to the rescue when family or friends needed help, but now they are the ones asking for assistance.

"I had to get comfortable with that," she said.

While DBS surgery may not be a cure-all for every Parkinson's symptom or patient, it can help some for a time. Still, there are other avenues a sufferer can take to improve their quality of life.

Chapter 6:
Acceptance

Jose Blanco didn't walk into the Southeast Volusia Family YMCA in Edgewater, he shuffled. With his feet lifting barely an inch off the floor and moving only a fraction more forward with each step, the 81-year-old New Smyrna Beach resident leaned on a cane for support, his once six-foot, two-inch tall body contorted into a stooped, comma-like shape.

A native of Spain, Jose came to the United States when he was 8 years old, living much of his life in New York City. He earned a bachelor's and master's degree in electrical engineering from City College of New York before moving to Massachusetts where he spent his professional career as a systems engineer.

"I have had Parkinson's disease for almost 20 years," Jose said while resting before an exercise class.

His journey with the disorder began when his wife noticed a twitching in his finger during dinner. Realizing this was not normal, she scheduled an appointment with a doctor, he said.

"He said right away that I had Parkinson's," Jose recalled. "I didn't know anything about the disease and was afraid what the repercussions would be."

Still, he decided to make the best of his circumstances.

"I came to the realization there was only so much I could do, and the thing to do was be as happy as I could," he said. This attitude served him well.

That, however, does not mean Jose took a passive approach toward the chronic disorder. He said not only did he go see the head of the neurology department at Boston University for advice, but he also participated in clinical trials of medications designed to treat Parkinson's.

Jose said it was the kind of testing where a patient gets a pill, but they don't know what kind of pill—a placebo or the test medication.

"Nothing came of it as such," he said of the trials.

Jose, who has taken Sinemet, the brand name for carbidopa/levodopa, for his symptoms for almost two decades, said the cynic in him sometimes suspects the pharmaceutical companies haven't discovered a cure for Parkinson's because they know they have a steady source of income from the drugs used to treat its symptoms.

"It has been a little discouraging," he said of the lack of progress toward ending the disease.

Jose said, in its early stages, Parkinson's really didn't have much of an impact on his life. The disorder never kept him from achieving any of his career goals, such as becoming a director of engineering for a major aerospace company. He was also able to spend time with his seven grandchildren and travel throughout Europe with his wife. But eventually the degenerative ailment took its toll.

"I loved playing tennis, and I had to give that up," he said. "That is something that I lost due to Parkinson's."

And as the disorder progressed, so did the limitations it caused.

"One of the most annoying symptoms is the lack of balance," Jose said. There is also the freezing, (stopping suddenly while walking), as he tries to go through narrow doorways. "I have to push myself to get moving again."

In addition to his issues, Jose said he feels badly for his spouse of 58 years, Maria Teresa, because of the way his Parkinson's has affected her.

"She was always there when I needed her. She treated it like it is was a normal thing and did not baby me," he said. "I am glad she behaved the way she did."

Sitting in the living room of the couple's waterfront New Smyrna Beach condominium, Maria Teresa said Jose's Parkinson's impacted her from the beginning.

"It was a shock," she said of her husband's diagnosis. "I felt so bad for him. I knew there was no cure, only medication to control the symptoms."

Maria Teresa said Jose's ailment initially allowed the couple to live as they planned. When Jose retired from the aerospace industry, they moved to a small community on the Massachusetts coast where he took a job in real estate. They built their dream house, a three-story structure on the water, that allowed for visits from the grandchildren during the summers. The couple also traveled and spent the winters in Florida.

But eventually, Jose's loss of mobility forced them to trade their dream home for a condominium with an elevator instead of stairs; the trips became more infrequent as well.

"It has been a total change," said Maria Teresa of their lifestyle. For example, the couple, whose love affair started in a New York City dance hall, found they could no longer dance.

"There is no intimacy," she said of the relationship with her husband. "I have to sleep in a separate bedroom because he thrashes his arms at night when he sleeps, and sometimes I have trouble understanding him because he slurs his words."

According to Maria Teresa, there have been cognitive changes as well. She said Jose suffers memory lapses and side effects from his medications, such as hallucinations.

"He does not realize that it is hard on me," she said.

Even simple tasks like emptying the dishwasher or making the bed became points of conflict for the couple, because while Jose wants to do these chores, Maria Teresa says it was easier for her to do them herself.

"I let him do them, so he can feel like he is helping," she said.

Maria Teresa added, Jose is not always realistic about Parkinson's toll on him.

"A couple of years ago, he said, 'maybe I will get better.' He is not going to get better."

There are times, she says, when her patience reaches its limits.

"It is like a prison sentence," she said of the daily challenges of being a Parkinson's caregiver. "Sometimes I feel like walking out and leaving, although I will never do that."

Maria Teresa acknowledges there have also been some positive results from Jose's illness, like the softening of certain elements of her husband's personality. The product of a frugal, farming family, she said Jose was always cautious with money and that was a point of conflict during their marriage. But he has eased up a bit as his Parkinson's has progressed.

"I think he is trying to compensate. He is trying to keep me happy and keep me around," she quipped. "I also feel he loves and appreciates me more."

Maria Teresa and Jose may have faced his Parkinson's from different sides of the same coin, but it was a challenge they took on together until Jose's death in May 2014.

Chapter 7:
Lab Rat

One of the most direct ways a patient can be involved in their Parkinson's treatment is by participating in clinical trials and research studies, or by becoming what I like to call "a lab rat."

The patient may be asked to do something as simple as tapping their thumb and index finger together or opening and closing their hand as fast as they can or touching a finger in front of them then touching their own nose or stomping a heel up and down on the floor.

What do such seemingly innocuous exercises have to do with Parkinson's? In the summer of 2014, Dr. Nawaz Hack and Dr. Umer Akbar were using data collected by observing patients performing these activities to better the lives of deep brain stimulation (DBS) therapy recipients.

The pair, working with principal investigator Dr. Michael Okun at the Center for Movement Disorders and Neurorestoration at the University of Florida, were testing six software updates to see if any would provide longer battery life of DBS pulse-generators developed by Medtronic Inc. To find out which pattern worked the best, the researchers had to have volunteers with Medtronic generators implanted in them.

Since I had such a device placed in the left-side of my chest in 2013 after my second deep brain stimulation surgery, the day before my annual generator check-up, I received a call asking that I participate in the study. I also had a Medtronic pulse-generator implanted during my first DBS procedure in 2011, but it was an older model and could not be reprogrammed.

Volunteers agreed to have their devices turned off and endure the return of tremors, slowness and rigidity, while the researchers inputted the temporary software updates. The purpose was to see which of the updates reduced the generator's battery output, while still controlling the patient's symptoms.

Meeting with Dr. Hack and Dr. Akbar at the appointed time, I was led to an empty conference room in the four-story building that houses the Center for Movement Disorders.

This Mutt and Jeff pair explained what they were going to do and what they hoped to learn before having me sign a waiver giving my permission to be reprogramed, videotaped, and the test data eventually disseminated.

Dr. Akbar told me I would be identified only as Subject 6, as I was the sixth person to undergo the testing. He then laid the programmer across my left shoulder, its sensor lining up with the pulse-generator in my chest, and inputted the first settings for voltage, duration and frequency.

"Say, 'today is a sunny day'," Dr. Akbar instructed, before he asked me to perform the series of exercises. Upon completion of this routine, he manipulated my head, neck and arms, checking my body's stiffness as Dr. Hack videotaped the entire process.

Dr. Hack then instructed me to follow him out of the room and to a corridor behind the center's patient check-in area. There, a young assistant recorded my gait as I walked across a pad connected to a computer.

This went on for about four hours. Each step was repeated precisely as a new program was inputted. When we were finished, Dr. Akbar informed me that three of the test programs seemed to reduce my battery's output before he restored my generator's original settings.

Why do it?

Participating in research like the Medtronic study gives a patient the chance to be part of discovering new ways to slow or stop the progression of Parkinson's; however, being a test subject, or "lab rat," can come with risks. Sometimes a person is recruited to try a new drug or therapy that does not work. This was the case during one clinical trial I volunteered for in 2008. I was one of more than 1,700 people asked to take part in a five-year, double-blind study that delved into what possible effect the nutritional supplement creatine might have on Parkinson's disease.

It was believed creatine could improve the function of the mitochondria, a cell's energy engine, and possibly act as an antioxidant, thus preventing damage caused by compounds harmful to brain cells.

However, when the Journal of the American Medical Association published the results of this trial in 2015, it concluded that, of the patients with early and treated Parkinson's disease, those who took creatine for at least five years showed no clinical improvement over those treated with a placebo.

I do not, nor will I ever, know whether I received the supplement or the placebo prior to my withdrawal from the trial to undergo deep brain stimulation surgery in 2011. Yet by participating, I have to believe that some good may have come from being poked, prodded and asked to pee in a cup in the name of science.

Timing can be important in trials as well, because once a patient begins a treatment regimen or undergoes deep brain stimulation therapy, they may no longer meet the research study criteria.

Not all studies deal with drugs. During a recent conference in Tampa, I was approached to see if I was interested in participating in a project that studied whether playing the piano has any cognitive, motor and psychosocial effects on Parkinson's disease.

Research may not always benefit a test subject directly, but the information it provides can help the Parkinson's community as a whole. Without volunteers, researchers cannot determine if a new treatment is safe or effective. And while not everyone has the financial resources to establish a non-profit foundation whose goal is to find a cure for Parkinson's, like Michael J. Fox, even a middle-aged journalist from a small town in Central Florida can answer a few survey questions, give a little blood or walk down a hallway in order to expand our knowledge.

Paying it forward

Like a pickpocket, Parkinson's disease sneaks up on its victims and robs them, not of their money, but of their independence. As it progresses, this degenerative condition can make even the simplest tasks, like getting out of bed, getting dressed, or driving to the store for groceries, insurmountable obstacles to those who suffer from it. This is why I believe in "paying it forward."

This philosophy is a belief that by helping others while expecting nothing in return, a person builds positive karma and someday someone will come to their aid in their time of need.

Such reciprocation can take any form; from lending someone a hand with their groceries to contributing money to a favorite charity.

My parents taught me to offer a helping hand at an early age.

We were on a family road trip and had stopped at a service plaza on the Florida Turnpike. Being a typical pre-teen, I ran into the building ahead of some woman, not thinking to hold the door open for her or let her enter ahead of me. My father was so outraged by such rudeness from one of his sons that he made me stand at the door for the next 15 minutes, opening it for everyone wishing to enter or exit the building. I was mortified, but the lesson worked, and to this day, I still open doors and allow people to go ahead of me.

One might say this is just good manners, but all a person has to do is watch as someone using a walker or in a wheelchair tries to navigate a closed door to know how much such consideration is needed, if not always extended.

Lending a helping hand does not have to extend just to Parkinson's sufferers to benefit from positive karma. For several years, I mowed the lawn next to my Edgewater home. This started one afternoon when I saw my elderly neighbor, Jack, on his knees trimming his lawn with a pair of hedge clippers. I had tried to cut his grass in the past but was run off by Jack. He told me that he was letting his lawn grow so it would seed some bare spots in his yard. This time was different, however. When I offered to mow his sod, Jack wanted to know if I wanted something in return. I said no, so he accepted my offer.

I looked at this service as neighbor helping neighbor and thought of the hour or so it took to push my lawnmower over his corner lot as part of my exercise routine.

When Jack died, and his son inherited the house, my lawn service continued for a time, although I was compensated occasionally with a bottle of Jack Daniel's whiskey.

Speaking of exercise and philanthropy, in the fall I usually join a couple hundred other Parkinson's sufferers, their caregivers and the able-bodied in walking around a Port Orange lake for the annual Parkinson's Association of Greater Daytona Beach's Sole Support fun walk to raise money to fight the disorder. And recently I became a volunteer "cornerman" for the local Rock Steady boxing affiliate in my area.

Admittedly, I have selfish motives for these acts. I want to prove to others, but mostly to myself, that I am still physically capable of performing such tasks.

For 30 years, I toiled day after day to produce a story or photographs for whatever publication employed me. My identity and self-worth were tied to my name in the byline above an article or in the credit-line under a photograph I had taken. Then Parkinson's robbed me of the physical and mental ability to do my job on a daily basis.

Now, more than five years into my forced retirement, I have come to the conclusion that Parkinson's disease isn't some conspiracy concocted to make me feel useless. Instead, it has provided me with insight into a life that I likely would have never encountered without it. It opened my eyes to the fact the world can change in an instant and you have to change with it or be left behind.

Chapter 8:
Deal with It

When I was told I had Parkinson's disease, a dark cloud settled over me and my mind was filled with questions. What kind of husband could I be to Beverly? Could I work with this disorder? Would I be able to get health insurance?

The more questions I asked, the darker my mood became.

Why did this happen to me? I am not anyone special, just a middle-aged, work-a-day journalist with a penchant for photography and fly-fishing. If this was somebody's idea of a bad joke, I was not laughing.

Despite having the emotional support of family and friends, I would only speculate on the negative aspects of my situation. I saw myself aging beyond my years. My 6-foot, 2-inch tall frame shuffling slowly behind a walker, hunched into the shape of a quotation mark with muscles so stiff I couldn't reach the bathroom in time to prevent an embarrassing accident.

Some of these predictions have come true. My feet drag when I walk, I have experienced memory loss and I am told there is a muffling of my usually boombox-like voice.

I also awaken most mornings to a body with the rigidity of a wooden plank, while at the same time possessing a steadiness of foot that rivals the pitching deck of a small boat on a wind-tossed sea.

Unfortunately, I am not alone in this struggle. Beverly is an emotional, if not physical, casualty of this neurological disaster, too. She has become so consumed with the effects Parkinson's disease has had on me that she says she can no longer separate the two. She even went so far as to say the man she married more than a quarter-century ago, no longer exists.

"You are not as outgoing as you once were. You used to be the first one to tell a story, now you are more in a shell," Beverly once told me, adding there are times I seem to zone out completely when we are with other people.

She has also changed. Evolving from a wife into more of a caregiver. This is something she sees as a positive.

"Maybe that is because I feel I am better at that," Beverly said. "But I am not going to baby you."

Beverly's first reaction to the news that I had Parkinson's was, "we'll deal with it."

Now she focuses so much of her attention on caring for me that sometimes it seems like she no longer trusts me to care for myself. She constantly reminds me to make sure I am carrying my medications with me when I leave the house, and that I take them on schedule. At the same time, she urges me to "be careful" as I trip over my own feet.

This can get old after a while, but there is a basis for her concern; especially considering my "if it isn't obviously causing a problem, then I don't need to worry about it" attitude toward my health.

More and more I find myself depending on Beverly to keep me on the right path. But is this fair to her? Shouldn't I be adult enough to deal with my own situation? After all, 25 years ago when we vowed to love and support each other for better or for worse, that didn't mean Beverly should get the short end of the stick all the time. She didn't count on this disease any more than I did, and I shouldn't expect her to put up with my angry outbursts and tantrums when things don't go my way.

Parkinson's may have aged me beyond my years, but it hasn't given me the right to turn into a grumpy old man.

I hope, that by recognizing these faults, I may have taken a step in the right direction toward fixing them. A path that represents a mellowing of my "glass is half-empty" mindset. Although, to say I'm now an optimist, might be going a bit too far.

Refusing to Succumb

I attribute this glimmer of hope to my fellow Parkinson's sufferers.

Even after witnessing the ravages our shared disorder has inflicted on many of them, I find most continue to have an air of optimism as they carry on their daily lives. These are people who refused to succumb to Parkinson's destructiveness and continue to fight what some might say is a losing battle against it.

This positive attitude could not have been better illustrated than when I watched one of my

"Dance for PD" classmates run from one end of our exercise room to the other.

Normally, this elderly gentleman named Mark, who has since passed away, could barely stand or move from place to place without assistance. But there he was, following our leader as she encouraged us to pick up our feet and run. Admittedly, he had his wife on one side and an aide on the other helping him along, but he still surprised us all with his effort. The room filled with joy and applause as he settled into a chair to catch his breath.

Watching such examples has made me recognize that having and keeping a positive attitude can be as valuable as medication in dealing with Parkinson's. It won't stop the tremors or freezing, but focusing only on the negative can lead a person to the conclusion that life is not worth living, and the consequences of that can be devastating. On the other hand, concentrating on the positives provides a motivation to live life to its fullest.

Helga is a Parkinson's sufferer who subscribes to this latter belief.

"I think life is good," she said while waiting for our exercise class to begin.

When asked how she maintains her positive outlook, the New Smyrna Beach resident said her secret is staying busy. "That way I am not moping around the house feeling sorry for myself."

I try to reflect a similar "can-do" attitude in dealing with my Parkinson's, but that is a trick I have not quite mastered yet. This is when I count on Beverly to drag me back from whatever has gotten me down.

"Deal with it," is her usual unspoken response when I complain about something. This is quickly followed by an equally silent "and fix it," which is her way of telling me to stop feeling sorry for myself.

In short, we Parkinson's sufferers need to live by the motto: When life hands you lemons, get out the juicer, limes, tequila and salt and make margaritas.

Learn to laugh

One way we can shake this negativity is by laughing, or so said certified laughter leader Diane Trask, as the dark-haired woman urged dozens of people attending a meeting of the

Parkinson's Association of Greater Daytona Beach, to repeat after her.

"Ho, ho, ho. Ha, ha, ha. Yeaaah!" she said.

Her audience echoed her cadence, then broke into its own guffaws, giggles and general merriment.

"Laughter is very contagious and it is free," Trask said.

This physiological response to watching the "Three Stooges" or listening to George Carlin's "Al Sleet, the Hippie, Dippy, Weatherman," also promotes positive physical and mental health, Trask said as she introduced the group to Laughter Yoga, an exercise and wellness program, created by Indian physician Dr. Madan Kataria.

According to the Laughter Yoga website, what began in 1995 with just five people in a park, has since grown to 6,000 laughter clubs in 60 countries around the world.

Laughter Yoga involves laughing continuously for 15 to 20 minutes with short breaks of yogic breathing. And while laughter is not the same as humor, Dr. Kataria discovered there is no difference in terms of the health benefits between pretend and genuine laughter.

(A brief History of Laughter Yoga and How it Originated, www.laughteryoga.org, Laughter Yoga International.)

"There is strong evidence that laughter can fight disease," Trask said. It has been shown to lower blood pressure, increase vascular flow and oxygenation of the blood, both of which can assist in healing. Laughter can also reduce stress hormones and increase infection-fighting antibodies, but it does not stop there.

"Laughter is exercise," the community liaison for Florida Hospital Hospice in Ormond Beach told the group. "Isn't that amazing."

Trask said laughter consists of two parts; a set of gestures and the production of sound. During the act of laughing, she said our brain pressures us into conducting both activities simultaneously. When people laugh heartily, as they did when they were children, changes occur in many parts of the body. Arm, leg and trunk muscles can be used until they ache, and, under certain circumstances, laughter can also cause the body to perform what the Encyclopedia Britannica describes as "rhythmic, vocalized, expiatory, and involuntary actions." Fifteen facial muscles contract and the epiglottis half closes the larynx so the intake of oxygen becomes irregular, causing a person to gasp, which sometimes makes their face turn red or purple.

Citing research that concluded laughing 100 times a day is equal to 10 minutes on a rowing machine or 15 minutes on an exercise bicycle, Trask even went so far as to call laughter a "full body, aerobic workout; all while sitting in your chair."

"It burns calories?" one audience member asked. "That is awesome."

Trask added that just by putting a smile on your face for three minutes, a person can change how they feel. Although looking around the room, I determined that smiling just for the sake of smiling can also make a person appear a bit mad.

Trask concluded her presentation by taking the audience on a mental journey that demonstrated how a person can use their imagination to contribute to this positive process. She invited everyone present to join her on what she called "a laughter roller-coaster."

We "hee, hee, hee 'ed" our way up an imaginary incline, "ho, ho, hoo'ing" our way back down again. Then we wriggled and giggled to imaginary ants in our pants.

Laughter is Universal

So, how does a person use laughter to deal with Parkinson's disease? I got an answer to that question thanks to email correspondence from the other side of the world sent by certified Laughter Yoga teacher and chair yoga trainee Roger David Borrow.

Borrow, a native of Australia now living in Singapore, specializes in helping and inspiring people with mobility problems to live happier, healthier lives by making them laugh.

A Parkinson's sufferer himself, Borrow said he understands how it feels to have normal day-to-day activities taken away by the disorder.

While his peers call him an inspiration and Singapore's biggest contributor to the Parkinson's cause, Borrow said his purpose is much simpler.

"When I teach a Laughter Yoga class, it gives me a sense of well-being and lifts my spirits. At first, I thought it was some sort of a scam because of the name, but once I attended a class, I was hooked. Now I try to laugh every day," he said

Borrow says laughter yoga has also had an impact on his emotional wellbeing and how he views his own Parkinson's.

"It keeps me positive and gives me self-worth by doing positive things for others," he wrote in his emails.

According to the Parkinson's Disease Society Singapore (PDSS), since being diagnosed in 2009, Borrow has refused to succumb to Parkinson's.

Rather than retreating into himself, he retired from his job as a production manager in the graphic arts industry and went on a two-month sailing voyage to Northern Australia. He invited his wife, Catherine, to join him and they spent another three weeks sailing around the Whitsunday Islands.

He also enjoys selecting and preparing dinner recipes for his spouse and likes to travel with her on business trips, "cherishing any and all opportunities to learn about and understand various cultures."

Borrow has taught classes combining laughter and exercise in Australia, India and

Singapore. Not only have these sessions received glowing reviews from participants and fellow teachers alike, but they also won Borrow the sixth annual Parkinson's Disease Society of Singapore's Star Award for his contribution to Parkinson's disease in 2013. The World Parkinson's Program also honored Borrow with its Dr. Rana International Parkinson's Community Service Award for his volunteer contributions to Singapore's Parkinson's groups.

The World Parkinson's Program is a global ideological movement whose mission is to improve the lives of those affected with Parkinson's disease, directly or indirectly. Its aim is to reach every individual across the world who has been affected with Parkinson's disease and educate them in their native tongue, as well as provide other support services. Founded in 2008 under a central theme that "those who fight Parkinson's with knowledge always find solutions," the program has chapters across the globe.

Its central executive committee annually honors up to three outstanding individuals who are committed to improving the quality of life of people with PD. The tireless dedication and hard work of such individuals not only makes a difference in the quality of life of those with the disease, but also helps caregivers better cope with the stress and ease the burden of taking care of their loved ones. (World Parkinson's Program)

Closer to home

Like Borrow, Linda Marlow said she gets as much out of teaching laughter classes as her participants seem to get from taking them.

"When I come out of a session, it feels like I am walking two feet in the air," the 70-something Ormond Beach, Florida resident said.

A professional ballroom dancer, who once owned her own dance studio in Miami, Marlow has been a laughter leader and instructor since 2002. She teaches laughter sessions to a variety of groups in the Daytona Beach area.

"Laughter is a stress reliever," she said. "Everyone has stress; even a person with perfect health, with a gazillion dollars in the bank and with a perfect family. Even when everything is perfect, people have stress in their lives. You can have stress just by turning on the television or driving in traffic."

Marlow said such stress lowers a person's immune system and laughter can help build it up again.

Marlow tells a story about a man who attended one of her classes in Miami. She said he suffered both physical and emotional problems related to his Parkinson's disease.

After the class, a woman came up to Marlow and identified herself as the man's psychologist. Marlow said the woman told her after just that one class, she could see a difference in her patient, saying he was happier and more socially outgoing.

"She said, 'You reached him when I couldn't'," Marlow recalled. "That is very rewarding."

According to Marlow, laughter provides other tangible benefits as well. Describing it as "inner-jogging," she said laughter releases "good chemicals" into the brain and body, such as serotonin, that can act as pain relievers.

Marlow says she has students who tell her that they started a class with a headache, but by the time it was over, their pain was gone. She added, while she forces no one to partake in her classes, it is not unusual for even nonparticipants to be laughing by the end of a session.

More to it.

Sometimes it takes more than a positive attitude or laughter to battle the negative effects of Parkinson's. Sometimes you have to build a foundation from which to fight. That is exactly what retired professional basketball star Brian Grant did after learning he had the disease.

The veteran of the National Basketball Association, who played for five different teams during his 12-year career, and I met in the spring of 2017 when he spoke at a conference in Orlando.

Grant said his body began telling him something was wrong, from the perspective of Parkinson's, as his career was winding down at the age of 36.

"I started noticing things like I could no longer jump off my left leg, which is my dominant leg," he said.

Speaking to an audience of about 500 in a ballroom at the Altamonte Springs Hilton hotel, Grant recalled the fear he experienced upon learning of his diagnosis.

"It was very scary," the Portland, OR, resident said. "The only thing I knew about Parkinson's was from what I had seen observing Michael J. Fox and Muhammad Ali."

Grant said he began asking himself questions like, "I am 6-foot, 9-inches (tall). If I am like that (off balance and suffering a constant tremor), how am I going to function? How am I going to live?"

But that wasn't his biggest concern. What bothered him the most was that nobody could tell him what he could do about his Parkinson's.

"Not even my neurologist, who is one of the top neurologists in the country and sits on the Michael J. Fox Foundation board."

He said it was for that reason he wasn't willing to open up about his illness in the beginning. "I didn't know if I wanted the whole world to know about it."

Eventually, Grant said it was questions from the youngsters he coached on his son's youth basketball team that prompted him to break his silence.

"They asked, 'Mr. Grant, Why is your hand shaking?'" he said.

Those queries, along with telephone calls from Michael J. Fox and Muhammad Ali's widow, Lonnie, asking that he join the Parkinson's fight convinced Grant to take action.

According to a video of a meeting between Fox and Grant that was broadcast on the Brian Grant Foundation website, the actor, who is barely tall enough to reach the basketball player's waist, told Grant that he had been given the challenge of Parkinson's because he was big enough to take it on."

"When a person is faced with such a burden, ...You don't pray for a lighter load, you pray for broader shoulders. And you have the broadest shoulders I have ever seen," Fox told the basketball star. (Brian Grant Foundation)

But it was his conversation with Lonnie Ali, Grant said, that truly prompted him to turn his diagnosis into something positive. He said Lonnie Ali urged him to not only take up the Parkinson's fight, but fight to win. That is when he decided to make it his personal mission to ensure those impacted by Parkinson's have the support system they need and the knowledge that they are not alone. This became the purpose behind the Brian Grant Foundation.

"Its mission is to serve as an inspirational and informational resource, helping individuals impacted by Parkinson's live active and fulfilling lives," Grant said. The Brian Grant foundation provides affordable exercise programs, wellness retreats, nutritional resources, community building and more. Each element is based on research and the expertise of some of the top people in the Parkinson's field, he said

This walking wall of a man doesn't just talk the talk, he has made himself a living example of his foundation's philosophy that a person can not only live with Parkinson's disease, but thrive with it.

To illustrate this point, Grant spoke of achieving two of his personal goals, learning how to skateboard and surf, after his diagnosis. He also talked about climbing Mount St. Helens with six other Parkinson's sufferers.

"Parkinson's disease is not a death sentence," Grant said.

Chapter 9:
Coming face to face

To paraphrase singer/songwriter Harry Chapin: *I have gone from "feeling all of 45 going on 15" to the far more realistic, "feeling all of 57 going on 80."*

I came to this truth a couple of years ago when Beverly and I were asked to help our son Brian and his family relocate into a new home in Jacksonville. Not only did my Parkinson's have me tripping over my own feet, but I didn't have the strength needed to keep my end up as we maneuvered furniture into place.

During my senior year in high school, I worked at a home decor store where part of my job was to deliver clients' purchases. At that time, I would think nothing of carrying a dining room table up the steps of a house or setting up a dresser in an upstairs bedroom. But, almost four decades later, I could barely keep pace with Brian as we carried his family's possessions from one abode into another. And by the time we had finished, I was moving like a rusty tin man.

One might say, as Beverly did while we were driving home, "when we were Brian's age (in his mid-30s) we would not have given such exertions a second thought."

That is no longer the case, however. While I know my body no longer possess the abilities it did 30 or 40 years ago, I don't want to solely blame age for this loss. To do so would mean I am consciously letting go of my youth, and that is something I am not prepared to do quite yet.

I may be pushing 60 in calendar years, but I want to believe I am still the same person I was in my 20s; hopefully a bit more experienced. Parkinson's, however, has me feeling and performing like I am in my 80s or maybe even older.

When I commented on this to Brian, after we carried half of a dining room curio cabinet into the house and had to stop twice to rest in the 50-yard distance between my pick-up and its final resting place, he was kind enough to say how impressed he was with my physical abilities, despite his bearing the majority of the load.

There are other signs Parkinson's has taken its toll that I find hard to accept. My fly cast, never as efficient as I would like it to be, has become less smooth and coordinated as I find it harder to get my arms to work in concert. And we won't even talk about lifting myself out of a kayak after a fishing trip. I also find myself looking at the walking stick standing in the corner of my bedroom, wondering if this is the day I will need its support.

The clock marches on.

I know having Parkinson's disease means I'm not the man I once was, but that does not mean I am ready to quit fighting yet. I still want to continue to enjoy all life has to offer for as long as possible.

When I was first diagnosed with the disease, it had little, if any, impact on my daily life. But over the past decade, I have become increasingly aware of the toll Parkinson's has taken on me.

Activities that once required little or no effort now require advanced planning. Something as simple as rising from our family room couch now dictates that I be aware of my lack of balance and a weakening of my legs, lest my upward thrust may turn into an awkward tumble backward. Pulling on a pair of pants used to be a one leg after the other while standing proposition, but no more. Now such casualness inevitably ends with a tumble into the clothes hanging in my closet. Even putting on a pair of shoes means grabbing an ankle and forcing my foot high enough to slip my toes past the heel of my sneakers. And if that isn't enough, a lack of attention toward how I might be leaning at the moment I bend down to tie my shoelaces can result in an embarrassing spill or kicking Johnny Cash, the family dog, in the face (which leads to a recriminating "what did I do wrong" look from the friendly pooch).

I can no longer easily get down onto one knee to compose a photograph with an upward angle, nor climb on a chair to change a light bulb. The steadiness I once possessed is gone, replaced with something akin to a baby taking its first steps.

Still, I have learned a valuable lesson over the years. Use caution, make the most of what you have, be grateful for it and never take anything for granted; for once you lose the ability to do something, you have to work twice as hard to regain it.

Chapter 10:
Let's Get Physical

Turning left out of the elevator and walking into the fourth-floor patient waiting area of the Center for Movement Disorders and Neurorestoration at the University of Florida a few years ago, I noticed a photograph hanging on the wall. It was the picture of a woman with an expression of rapture on her face, her arms spread wide and her body a blur of fluid motion. A person might question the appropriateness of such an image being displayed in a setting where most of the persons waiting to be seen are confined to wheelchairs, move with hesitant steps, shuffle behind a walker or lean on a cane for support. But there was a sense of hope in this photograph.

One of the most likely first questions a newly diagnosed Parkinson's patient will ask their physician is, "How do I slow the progression of this chronic condition?"

Notice I said slow, not stop, the physical and mental deterioration that accompanies Parkinson's disease. To date, there is nothing known to medical science that can cure this affliction; however, there are steps a patient can take to turn the downward spiral of Parkinson's from a free fall to a controlled tumble. One of the simplest is exercise.

A Profanity

Before being diagnosed more than a dozen years ago, the word "exercise" was an eight-letter profanity in my pre-Parkinson's vocabulary.

I was more than 30 pounds overweight and the only workout I got was chasing my grandchildren around the house while trying to convince them it was time to go down for a nap. The nap wasn't for them, it was for me.

Post-diagnosis, my doctors encouraged me to take up some form of regular physical activity in the spirit of continued movement. And when that didn't work, there were dire predictions of what could happen if I choose to ignore their advice.

Still, I continued my sedentary lifestyle even after watching the group represented by the photograph. They were members of a "Dance for Life" group, who performed during a

2009 Parkinson's symposium I attended at the University of Florida in Gainesville. These dancers moved with grace and rhythm despite the limitations Parkinson's had placed upon them.

When asked if I exercised on any regular basis, I would laugh nervously and come up with one excuse after another to justify my laziness. My fitness routine consisted of climbing the stairs rather than using the elevator at work; or slowly paddling my kayak across the waters of the Mosquito Lagoon and the Indian River in East Central Florida while fly fishing for redfish and/or sea trout. I would equate walking up to the second-floor newsroom at the News-Journal building or overcoming the influence of a tidal flow or gentle breeze while trying to cast a fly toward my lock-jawed quarry, with the effort it once took to propel my younger self across the rugby pitch at the University of Oregon.

In my early years with Parkinson's, work substituted for exercise. The mental and physical exhaustion I felt after putting in 40-plus hours a week as a newspaper reporter/photo-journalist became a convenient excuse for my lack of physical activity. But as my disorder progressed, I found gathering and disseminating the news of the day to be not as easy as it had once been. There was a time when spending hours covering a story, then going back to the newsroom to write it on deadline was like mainlining adrenaline, and reporting on two or three events in a given day was just part of the job. Then Parkinson's robbed me not only of the ability to make such a contribution to the profession I loved, but also the desire to do so. My enthusiasm for getting the story was replaced by a pull of fatigue, and my output waned to the point I was no longer satisfied with the effort I was able to muster. "Robo-reporter" had become just another regular-reporter, and that wasn't good enough.

As luck would have it, about this same time, corporate downsizing in the newspaper industry led to the elimination of my position at the News-Journal. So, after 30 years of covering the news, I found myself out of a job, just two months shy of when I had decided to retire anyway due to the effects of my Parkinson's.

"This has nothing to do with performance," the paper's executive editor said repeatedly as he told me I was being laid off in

October 2013, seven years after I had been diagnosed. But when I look back on some of the articles I authored toward the end of my career, I suspect this was not entirely true; it was obvious I was not doing my best work.

While I do not miss the stress or the employment uncertainty that comes with the digitization of print journalism, I still feel a need to know what is going on when I drive past a police car parked outside a house, its blue lights flashing. I guess you can take the boy out of journalism, but not the journalist out of the boy.

Soon, I found hours once spent at a computer keyboard were replaced by the boredom of inactivity, and I quickly discovered I could spend only so much time sitting in front of the television. So, I began looking for an alternative means of whiling away my days.

Initially, this meant spending more time in the Mosquito Lagoon with fly rod in hand, fishing, but that crapped out when I discovered I could no longer haul myself from my kayak without assistance.

So, I returned to photography. Beverly had given me a modern digital camera to replace the one the News-Journal had supplied. I took a digital photography course at Daytona State College and then compiled years of Bike Week images into a book of portraits.

But both proved secondary to starting a regular exercise program.

Let the Exercise Begin

My road to physical fitness began with a semi-daily walk along the riverfront a couple of blocks east from my home. I would stroll down the sidewalk to a city park, a distance just far enough to generate a gleam of a perspiration across my forehead. I won't say sweat, because the exertion required to take this journey didn't merit such a description. Although when our family dog, a lab-mix mutt named Johnny Cash, joined me on these sojourns, I found keeping his 100-plus pounds of tail-wagging exuberance under control in between stops every few seconds to sniff the landscape, lift his rear leg or greet a fellow canine heading in the opposite direction, presented somewhat of a more physical challenge.

Soon these walks were combined with a series of short-lived (thanks to the wondrous limitations of the American medical insurance system) visits to a physical therapist. The therapist put me through an exercise program designed to improve my balance and counteract the body stiffness that comes with Parkinson's disease.

When my insurance-allotted number of therapy sessions ran out, a Wii video game console took the therapist's place and I began to exercise at home on my own. It was certainly much cheaper because, without insurance, each physical therapy appointment came with a price tag in the hundreds of dollars.

Eventually, I found a more social and cost-effective solution to my need for physical exertion. My balance and coordination were put to the test when Beverly and I joined a "Dance for PD" group.

Beverly encouraged my exercise efforts with the same enthusiasm she exhibited upon learning I had diabetes, which turned her into my very own "Diet Nazi;" scrutinizing everything I ate in the name of controlling my high blood sugar levels.

For someone who has been told he has no sense of rhythm, Dance for PD presented significant challenges. These "dance" classes consist of between two and 20 fellow Parkinson's sufferers and their caregivers who sit in a circle, flapping our arms and tapping our toes to the beat of the music. This is followed by a walk, march, slide or side-step around the oval with some participants using chairs for support, again keeping in time with the tunes. On other occasions, we tossed rubber balls or plastic hoops to one another (although catching these items seemed optional at best).

As this occurred, our instructor, a small Hispanic woman named Gabriela, used her heavily-accented voice to encourage her charges to hoot, holler and laugh, causing us to exercise our facial muscles and vocal cords as well. These actions might be followed by instructions to act out something from the world around us, like what a person might see during a trip to the circus or a journey on a boat; thereby giving our imaginations a workout too.

The vast majority of my fellow "dance class" participants are typical Parkinson's patients—people in their 70s or 80s, which led to a moment of self-discovery by the youngster of the group—me. Age does little to dampen enthusiasm.

Nothing is more motivating than being shown up by a woman old enough to be your mother as you try to keep pace with the instructor's commands. Equally as true, a personal lack of coordination is of little consequence when the person across the room from you may depend on a walker or a wheelchair, but still moves to the music with enthusiasm.

Giving his all

Maynard Kern provides just such a positive motivation. Although he is confined to a wheelchair much of the time, this 80-plus-year-old former owner of an air conditioning and heating business usually gives his all during our exercise classes.

This was not always the case, however. In the beginning, Maynard would sleep through much of the class, but the more engaged he became, the more he participated. Now he almost jumps from his chair so he can join the rest of us in exercising; a change that only took a few months. Such exuberance sometimes creates problems for Kern's wife, Arline, and his care-aide, lest he try to stand unexpectedly and fall.

"Maynard is a little bit different," Arline said, speaking for her husband, whose illness has robbed him of much of his voice. He could barely be heard above the background din as we sat in the lobby of Edgewater's Southeast Volusia Family YMCA.

Arline said her first clue something was wrong with her husband of 18 years, was a lack of expression on his face, along with a far-off stare. "His arms were also stiff when he walked, if they swung at all," she recalled. "The doctors say he has Parkinsonisms; a term referring to a group of neurological disorders that cause movement problems similarly to those seen in Parkinson's disease," Arline said. "Some days he is good and some days he is terrible. He can't even get himself out of a chair."

Still, Maynard has not allowed his frail physique to stop him from attempting to walk around the room or dance with his wife during our "Dance for PD" classes or punch the heavy bag during our Rock Steady boxing sessions.

Even though arthritis, a stroke, and Maynard's Parkinsonisms may limit his strength and range of motion, Maynard's never-say-die attitude continues to inspire all those around him; much like the smile that lights up his face when he is congratulated by his classmates for his efforts.

The Next Step

There is a saying in physics; "a body at rest tends to stay at rest, while a body in motion tends to stay in motion." Nowhere is this more true than with Parkinson's disease.

That is why Dance for PD became the root from which my oak of exercise grew. After a couple of years in the program, Gabriela suggested I expand my physical training, recommending I might benefit from one of the YMCA's "spin" classes. This aerobic endeavor calls for the participant to mount a stationary bicycle and pedal their way to fitness; an activity I naively thought would not be too strenuous for someone in my condition.

"If you want to be able to move tomorrow, you should just concentrate on keeping your legs moving," the spin instructor said during my first day in class as she demonstrated the standing, crouching and seated pedaling positions. I was expected to master these positions while keeping time with the rhythmic musical boom emanating from the stereo speakers on either side of the bicycle-filled room.

"It took me about a year before I could keep up," quipped a classmate, her feet rotating in a blur on the pedals of her bike.

For the next couple of months, I awoke twice a week and drove to the Y for an hour of pre-dawn pedaling. As my feet rotated the pedals of my bike, sweat poured out of me, soaking my clothes as I prayed my heart would not stop pumping oxygenated blood to the muscles required to keep my legs moving while I tried to keep pace with the rest of the class. In the end, it was my knee that gave out before my heart did.

Not all of my fitness efforts are as strenuous.

Beverly talked me into joining her in a "seated" yoga class. Here, a group of about two dozen senior citizens, mostly female, attempt to stretch muscles contracted through the passage of time into flexible fibers of elasticity and strength by twisting and bending our bodies in ways that would make a contortionist proud. We also work on balance by trying to stand on one leg and raising the opposite arm into the air while rising up on our toes; or put one foot in front of the other like a drunk driver taking a police field sobriety test.

This was soon followed, as part of the same Silver Sneakers senior fitness program as yoga, by my short-lived attendance in a class where elderly participants used rubber balls, elastic bands and small dumbbells to work up a minimal sweat, but that didn't offer enough of a challenge.

Seeking more "oomph!" in our workouts, Beverly and I joined a spin-off of our Dance for PD class called Power Moves!

This program is designed to provide its participants more than just exercise. It focuses on the practical applications of various body movements needed to perform such tasks as getting out of bed or standing after a fall. Participants lift and move their legs to the side of their chair just as a person does when getting out of a car. We focus on bringing a foot forward when we are on all fours, so we can brace ourselves to stand up.

I have also participated in "LSVT BIG" therapy. This encompasses 16 one-hour-long exercise sessions scheduled over a period of four weeks in which a participant performs a scientifically-researched series of exaggerated arm and leg movements under the watchful eyes of a certified therapist. While it does not have the socialization of Dance for PD, BIG does battle the tendency of Parkinson's patients to allow their bodies to withdraw inward; such as taking smaller steps or making smaller movements while thinking we are performing normally. This is why "BIG" participants are encouraged to continue the exaggerated steps, wide arm sweeps, and other such moves daily, for the rest of their lives.

Periodically, I also work out on my own. This effort consists of spending about an hour panting and grunting away on any of the variety of fitness machines in the Y's wellness center. These ellipticals, Stair-masters, rowing machines, weight-training devices and treadmills are designed to improve a person's physical fitness or, if some of the people exercising around me can be used as examples, at least create a sleek line of muscle-encased spandex.

My workouts usually begin with some time on a treadmill or the steps of an elliptical to get my heart pumping. And while I may not demonstrate the same enthusiasm as the woman running beside me, I am content to take a lazy stroll on the revolving rubber belt. This is followed by about 45-minutes of straining my way through various weight machines in hopes of enhancing my inner, if not my outer, self.

While I am not convinced of the aesthetic benefit of all this heavy breathing and muscle strain, there is a feeling of self-satisfaction when a total stranger remarks, "You look like you really worked hard today," as I walk sweat-stained out of the gym door.

Taking the fight to Parkinson's

Most recently, Beverly and I decided to take my battle with Parkinson's into the squared-circle when we joined a newly established affiliate of the national Rock Steady boxing program in our area.

Founded in 2006 by Marion County (Indiana) Prosecutor Scott C. Newman, who was diagnosed at the age of 40 with Young-Onset Parkinson's, Rock Steady is based on studies that suggest certain kinds of "forced" exercise might be neuroprotective, actually slowing the progression of Parkinson's. (Rock Steady Boxing.org)

These 90-minute, three-times-a-week sessions encourage participants to perform a variety of rigorous exercises that focus on pugilistic pursuits, but without the actual contact of combat.

Whether pounding a heavy bag with my fists, focusing on my footwork or jumping rope to the encouragement of our coaches will have any effect on my long-term Parkinson's prognosis, is still too early to tell. But I do know this, the program is kicking my ass.

Still, the infectious enthusiasm of coaches like Saturn "Animal" Robell, a 27-year-old yoga instructor by trade, go a long way toward making me and the approximately three dozen boxers enrolled at our gym forget our aches and pains and push ourselves a bit farther than we think we can go.

"I enjoy the sense of community Rock Steady creates," Saturn said before leaving the program to relocate to more northern locales. "It brings hope to so many people."

She said she has watched people enter the gym timid and unsure of what they are capable of, and in a short time they regain their self-confidence.

"I have been a healer my entire adult life," Saturn said. There is a remarkable difference between those she teaches without a life-altering, physically-limiting affliction and those who walk through the door at Rock Steady. "The latter boxers are fighting for their quality of life."

Another former coach and participant, Paul Boswell, who went by the boxing name of "Gator," couldn't agree more.

"It is a collaboration of things," the Parkinson's patient himself said of the benefits Rock Steady can achieve.

After two and a half years in the program, Gator said Rock Steady has not only helped with his confidence, but the physical exertion it promotes has reduced the pain and stiffness that accompany his Parkinson's. He said, in his opinion, Rock Steady is the only treatment from which he has truly benefited.

"The pills we take help with our symptoms," Gator said. "But boxing offers more. By giving back movement and balance, Rock Steady has helped improve my life."

That is exactly what Marianne Chapin said she had in mind when she started the Rock Steady (New Smyrna Beach) affiliate in early 2018. The local program has had its ups and downs in its first year in operation, like having to move twice before finding a home of its own in what was the gift shop of a former honey factory. Its participants have dedicated themselves to making the local affiliate work, giving both dollars and sweat to this to fight against Parkinson's disease.

Casting a Fly is an Exercise High

Not all exercise has to be done indoors. I found my love of fly fishing helps keep my body in motion, too.

For those who are unfamiliar with Robert Redford's cinematic endeavor "A River Runs Through It," fly fishing is the art of delivering an artificial lure—usually a bit of fur or feather tied to a small hook—in front of a fish with such delicacy that it will assume this manmade object is part of its natural predator/prey menu. Rather than the weight of the lure trailing a hair-thin strand of monofilament fishing line toward my query, the back-and-forth motion of the fly rod propels the line, which in turn carries the fly (lure) toward its target. This is accomplished when the fisherman performs a series of choreographed arm movements along with a shifting of body weight and center of balance.

Smoothness of motion is critical to successful placement of a fly, both in terms of distance and presentation. The rod arm moves along a parallel plane to the ground as its wrist cocks, giving the proper trajectory needed to lift the fly line off the water and throw it behind the fisherman in a tight loop as the rod loads or flexes. This generates the energy required to send the line and fly toward the fish as the casting arm moves the rod forward again. At the same time, the fisherman's non-rod hand grasps the fly line and "hauls" it back and forth generating additional speed, thus energy. While these actions take place, the angler focuses his or her attention on the ever-swimming target, while maintaining their balance on the sometimes-tricky footing of a slick algae, mud and rock-covered river bottom or wave-tossed boat deck. That doesn't take into account the chaotic frenzy created when the fish eats the fly, gets hooked and fights to free itself.

Multitasking at its finest!

Exercise may take many forms, but it is not the type of activity that matters. The lesson a Parkinson's patient must learn is if they don't want to become part of the furniture, then being a couch potato isn't an option.

Chapter 11:
Shaken, not Stirred

Within days of informing my family of my Parkinson's diagnosis, a package was delivered to my home via Federal Express from Amazon.com. It contained two books about the disorder, a gift from my brother Buck, the teacher.

This gift was motivated by the hope that I would educate myself about the disease and pass that information along to the rest of the family.

Since that day, education has been one key of many in dealing with my ailment, because the more a person knows about Parkinson's, the better equipped they are to deal it.

In addition to the books my brother sent: "Living Well with Parkinson's Disease" by Gretchen Garie and Michael J. Church, and "The First Year—Parkinson's Disease: An Essential Guide for the Newly Diagnosed" by Jackie Hunt Christensen; in the ensuing years, I have taken advantage of any number of educational resources to learn more about this chronic disease. I have attended conferences, listened to speakers, read other publications, addressed questions to Parkinson's "experts" and subjected myself to the poking and prodding of various research studies and clinical trials.

Compared to the average Joe on the street, it may seem like I'm an expert on the subject, but what I actually know is how little I understand about my illness. I may be able to explain the basic details of how Parkinson's disease affects the human brain and body. I can also describe what some treatments do and what it is like to suffer from some of the variety of symptoms it can produce; like tremors or what I call "the James Bond shaken, not stirred martini effect." When it comes down to the big question, "How do I get cured?" I am no closer to an answer than the aforementioned experts.

This is why we in the Parkinson's community must never stop learning. Every time we glean a new nugget of knowledge we take one more step on that long road toward a cure.

Back to the Future without Parkinson's

This is not a journey we can take alone. We must educate the Parkinson's sufferer and the non-sufferer alike, because the more interest our illness generates, the greater the attention it will be given.

This could not have been proven more true than when actor Michael J. Fox let it be known he suffered from Young-Onset Parkinson's disease.

Like it or not, when a person of public interest, such as a celebrity, becomes associated with a particular malady, this creates curiosity and more people want to know about that aspect of their lives.

Parkinson's affects approximately a million people in America and another 6 to 10 million worldwide annually, but little was said about it outside the Parkinson's community until it became the celebrity disease of the moment.

Fox initially hid his diagnosis from the glare of the public spotlight, as was his right. He said he would put his shaking hands in his pants pockets or hide an arm tremor by blocking it from view behind his body or part of a set.

It wasn't until he unveiled his private battle that interest in Parkinson's skyrocketed, fueling the general public's desire to learn more about the disorder. Fox added to this phenomenon when he founded the Michael J. Fox Foundation for Parkinson's Research, which has funneled millions of dollars into finding a cure for the disease.

In his memoir "Lucky Man," Fox credits Parkinson's with allowing him to take a different path on life's journey. He even went so far as to call it "unquestionably a gift."

"Nobody would ever choose to have Parkinson's disease visited upon them... but absent this neurological catastrophe, I would have never opened (the gift) or been so profoundly enriched," he said. (Lucky Man, Michael J. Fox, Hyperion, 2002, Page 5.)

Recognizing that most Parkinson's sufferers would not consider the disorder "a gift," the attention Fox has brought to the table through his foundation, books and a television special, unquestionably provides a gift of knowledge from which all Parkies can benefit.

But Fox is only one resource. There are hundreds of books available on the subject just as there are advocacy groups like the Parkinson's Action Network, the National Parkinson's Foundation, and the American Parkinson's Disease Association. Each of these organizations, and others like them around the world, provide up-to-date information about the latest medical research, hints on living with the disorder and how to address quality-of-life issues. It is up to the Parkinson's sufferer or their caregiver to seek them out.

Going to the Data

Beverly and I have learned much by attending such conferences, but the key to getting the most out of these events is keeping an open mind.

One example of this came about when we drove 111 miles north along Interstate 95 to the Mayo Clinic in Jacksonville to learn about Minor Cognitive Impairment (MCI). We initially planned to attend a discussion on Lewy-body dementia; a progressive decline in mental abilities that can present Parkinson's-like symptoms and Parkinson's disease, but it had been canceled. So, instead of going home, we went to the MCI talk under the assumption, wrongly as it turned out, that it would focus on cognitive issues associated with Parkinson's. Instead, it centered on dementia as it relates to Alzheimer's disease. Still, most of the topics discussed dovetailed nicely.

During one session, "What People Living with MCI and their Loved Ones Need to Know to Prepare for the Future," presenter Francine Parfitt talked of the importance of planning ahead. She spoke of the need for dementia patients to let their wishes be known on matters that may cause conflict in a time of medical catastrophe. These can include determining who holds financial and medical powers of attorney for the patient and if there is a do-not-resuscitate declaration. She also stressed the need for such decisions to be made while the patient is physically and mentally capable.

Parfitt, the co-director of the Outreach, Education, and Recruitment Core of the Mayo Clinic's Alzheimer's Disease Research Center in Florida, as well as director of the Memory Disorder Center and operations manager for Mayo Clinic Florida Neuroscience Clinical Research, emphasized a person can prepare all he or she wants, but if they do not let their wishes be known, they cannot be acted upon.

"This helps to ensure everyone understands your wishes," Parfitt said.

A colleague of Parfitt's, Dr. Nilufer Ertekin-Taner M.D., Ph.D., talked about Alzheimer's disease being a secondary problem for Parkinson's patients, but not an automatic one.

The neurologist and neurogeneticist offered a number of tips that may help keep the brain healthy. "Do all the things that are good for you," she said.

Some of her recommendations, like physical exercise and socialization, have proven to be beneficial for Parkinson's patients, as have other "healthy brain" activities including partaking in mental exercises such as reading, doing puzzles and/or learning something new. Taking vitamins, particularly B-complex and vitamin C, and getting quality sleep helps.

Diet is also important. Ertekin-Taner suggested eating fatty fish, wild salmon or mackerel for example, at least three times a week; consuming a handful of nuts daily; eating foods high in antioxidants or containing curry spice including cumin; and/or following a Mediterranean diet which includes red wine.

The National Parkinson's Foundation says the most common dietary concerns facing Parkinson's patients include bone thinning, dehydration, bowel impaction, un-planned weight loss and medication side effects—such as nausea, loss of appetite and/or compulsive eating.

Another nutrition-related concern Dr. Ertekin-Taner pointed out was the interaction in which levodopa competes with proteins in food for absorption through the small intestine. This requires a sufferer to pay attention to when they eat and when they take the drug. Generally, levodopa should be ingested at least a half hour before eating or two hours after a meal. (Parkinson's Disease: Nutrition Matters by Kathrynne Holden, M.S., R.D. National Parkinson's Foundation. Pages 2-3, 11-13.)

Dr, Ertekin-Taner's list also included treating cardiac risk factors like high blood pressure, diabetes, high cholesterol and being overweight. (Mayo Clinic, A Dozen Healthy Brain Tips.)

Her talk flowed into the final session of the day, stress management by Michelle Graff-Radford.

As with Parkinson's, she said stress can play a factor in Alzheimer's disease, and by reducing stress, a person can fight cognitive impairment.

"We all know life can be stressful. However, there are two critical elements that can directly impact how we experience stress," Graff-Radford said. "What we choose to focus our attention on and how we choose to interpret an event."

During her presentation, this slender woman with dark, shoulder-length hair and a gentle voice took the more than two dozen members in the discussion group through a series of stress management and relaxation techniques that included yoga, breathing, progressive muscle relaxation and Herbert Benson's Relaxation Method, which incorporates meditation.

Additionally, she spoke of how studies have shown practicing gratitude can make a person healthier and happier.

"Researchers have found people who regularly express their feelings of gratitude tend to experience less stress, have greater resistance to viral infections, sleep more soundly, have fewer physical complaints, spend more time exercising, and feel more optimistic," Graff-Radford said.

Whether the focus is about the latest research into the study of Alpha-synucleins or how to select an assisted living facility, the subject matter is not what is important. The crucial element is to never stop learning, and the simplest way to do that is through communication.

Chapter 12:
Spreading the Word

Upon learning of my diagnosis, I, like many other sufferers, was confronted with the question, "Do I tell others I have Parkinson's disease? And if so, how?"

Informing my family was a given as I could not hide my symptoms from those closest to me.

My wife, Beverly, accepted the news with a strength she has always shown in the face of adversity and has been by my side ever since.

She was scared, of course; not of becoming a caregiver, but of how I would cope with the emotional toll Parkinson's can have on a patient. I have little tolerance for frustration and a temper to match, so we both expected I would not deal well with the anticipated loss of voluntary motor control and the other physical symptoms that are mainstays of Parkinson's.

Unfortunately, in the years since my diagnosis, this prediction has proven true. I find I am less tolerant of many things, such as my lack of balance or the inability to make myself understood when I am talking to someone and I am quick to react badly to them. That's why I occasionally see a therapist to talk about how to deal with these and similar issues in a more productive way than just lashing out at those close to me.

After Beverly, the decision to inform my remaining kin wasn't as clear-cut. In 2006, my mother was battling lymphoma and her worry meter was about tapped out, so my father decided we should withhold my diagnosis from her. It was a decision for which we both suffered a rebuke when she learned of our deception.

As the news of my ailment spread to the rest of the family, I received expressions of concern and support. A niece asked my sister, "Is Uncle Mark going to be alright?"

While I assured her and others that I was going to be fine, at the time, I wasn't entirely confident of that myself.

Additionally, I faced the dilemma, "Do I tell anyone else?"

I had read that a person with such a condition should be careful about disseminating that information to his or her employer because it could be used against them. But I quickly discovered this is not always the case.

When I told the editors at the Daytona Beach News-Journal of my diagnosis, my immediate supervisor accepted the news without comment.

On the other hand, the newspaper's executive editor called me into his office. There he told me his father-in-law also suffered from Parkinson's and had gone to a specialist about the disorder.

He encouraged me to do the same thing because of the positive impact it had on his in-law's outlook about the disease.

This advice proved beneficial and I am grateful for the concern, which I would never have received if I hadn't put myself out there.

Putting the Word Out

I came out of the Parkinson's closet in early 2007 while attending a writing workshop at the Poynter Institute for Media Studies in St. Petersburg, Florida.

I was there for a work-related, week-long seminar entitled "Reporting and Writing the Untold Stories." The dozen or so seminar participants were tasked with writing an article on a subject personal to them, but not one they would necessarily talk about publicly. The resulting essays ranged in topic from an exploration of a person's ethnic background, the challenges of parenting as a single father, and alcoholism.

I wrote about my fear that Parkinson's might turn me from a relatively healthy, 46-year-old male into an "aging before my time, living bobble-head doll" and my concerns of how I might be perceived by others.

Shortly thereafter, I announced my diagnosis to the readers of the News-Journal in my column by saying I was on the receiving end of "one of life's curve balls."

For a time, in addition to covering my regular beats, I authored a weekly column that included subjects ranging from my reaction to the news of the day to family get-togethers. Parkinson's disease became just more column fodder.

Some people might say I was just looking for sympathy, but I saw these columns and the stories that followed as a way to educate my readers about this chronic disorder.

I wrote about all aspects of my Parkinson's—from its diagnosis to how I dealt with its symptoms and some of the treatments I had tried.

The reaction I received was an acceptance I could have never anticipated. Strangers and acquaintances alike read my words and responded via letters, phone calls and emails with a wide range of comments. Some readers told me they knew someone with Parkinson's, while others spoke about themselves, as was the case with a woman who approached me while I was working out at the gym.

I was standing between two weight-lifting machines when a lady in her 60s, walked up to me. After making sure she was talking to "the right Mark I. Johnson," the woman told me she was a fellow Parkinson's sufferer. We talked for several minutes before she thanked me for being so forthcoming about my Parkinson's. But it was I who was grateful for the courage she showed in opening herself up to me.

My columns opened other doors for me to talk about my experience with Parkinson's.

One such opportunity came in 2009 when I was invited to speak at the 7th annual

Parkinson's Disease Symposium, put on by the Center for Movement Disorders and Neurorestoration at the University of Florida.

In the beginning, I felt more than a little unqualified, sandwiched between one of the center's neurologists, Dr. Hubert Fernandez, and neurosurgeon Dr. Kelly Foote. I was at a loss as to what insights I might be able to provide that these Parkinson's experts wouldn't cover. That is when I decided to talk about a subject I knew about—how being open about my illness had positively affected my quality of life.

I told the symposium audience how being able to write about my Parkinson's had made dealing with the medication routine, the symptoms and the emotional toll easier by reducing the feelings of isolation that can accompany the disease.

One example I used was an incident when a woman came up to me in the grocery store and asked if she could give me a hug.

"I just wanted to tell you how much your Parkinson's stories mean to me," she said; although she did indicate she was not a Parkie herself.

When I finished my presentation, a woman walked up to the podium and thanked me for my candor. Specifically, she said, for my honesty about seeing a therapist to deal with the depression that Parkinson's can bring on. She said such insight gave her and others an example of courage that they could use in addressing the psychological impacts of the disorder.

According to the National Parkinson's Foundation, up to 50 percent of Parkinson's patients may experience some form of depression during the course of their illness. (Parkinson's Disease: Mind, Mood & Memory, Dan Weintraub M.D., National Parkinson's Foundation, 2007; page 7.)

It's just such comments that reinforce my decision to continue to speak openly about this affliction. I find this straightforwardness not only eases others' discomfort but benefits the sufferer too. By talking about their Parkinson's, the patient is afforded the position to ask and answer questions, discuss options and feel they have some control in what can appear to be an out-of-control situation.

Keeping Track

Another way to maintain control is to keep a Parkinson's journal, or so said Dr. Natalya Shneyder, a neurologist with University of Florida Health in Jacksonville.

This is something my wife has urged me to do for years so I won't be so dependent on her to remember things that might need addressing during doctor visits.

Dr. Shneyder, speaking to a meeting of the Parkinson's Association of Greater Daytona Beach, talked about the benefits of keeping track of the multitude of details related to the illness. When asked what should be included in such a journal, Dr. Shneyder said "anything that affects your quality of life."

She said these entries should represent the norm rather than the unusual, thus allowing a patient to present a factual picture of what happens to them on a daily basis. The Parkinson's Disease Society of the United Kingdom agrees. It suggests including data like how long you have had the disorder; what symptoms cause you the most problems; and details about your medications, like how many there are and how often you take them. It also suggested writing down medication specifications in one color ink and any problems you may have in another color. This way you and your doctor can tell, at a glance, if there is a connection between a problem or side effect and the medication. (Parkinson's Disease Society of the United Kingdom, London. Revised March 2008.)

Dr. Shneyder stressed that there is no need to record such detail every day. Instead, a patient should keep track of their data for just a few days prior to a doctor visit. This allows for an up-to-date record that can be shared without forgetting something. She also recommended entries be kept in half-hour increments, so your physician has a clear picture of the patient's day.

Sharing with Others

Support groups can be a beneficial tool.

These regularly scheduled gatherings of patients and/or caregivers not only provide an empathetic ear into which a Parkie can vent in a non-judgmental environment, but also offer a resource from which to discover something about the disorder they might have not otherwise considered.

I reached this conclusion while listening to 29-year-old Brandi Roman. She was a panelist during a Young-Onset Parkinson's conference Beverly and I attended in 2010. Roman received a standing ovation from a roomful of her fellow sufferers after relaying a tale of climbing Montana's highest peak through an August snowstorm. She said the trek was a way to prove to herself and others that while she had Parkinson's, it didn't have her.

"It was as though my diagnosis of Parkinson's put a mountain in my life's path," Roman told her audience. (Daytona Beach News-Journal.)

These stories tend to outshine the tales of ugliness about Parkinson's, but to hear them, a person needs to be willing to venture out and mingle with other Parkinson's disease sufferers.

This is one of the reasons why Beverly and I joined the Dance for PD exercise program in our area. On its face, this "dance class" is about staying mobile, but there's much more to it than toe-tapping or follow-the-leader to music.

Developed by the Brooklyn, NY-based Mark Morris Dance Group, the program offers

Parkinson's patients a judgment-free venue from which they can express themselves.

"The program is designed to provide folks with Parkinson's a way to explore movement and music in a safe, creative and positive environment," said David Leventhal of the Morris Dance Group. "Participants have told us that the class helps them feel more fluid and rhythmic in their movements and gives them a sense of confidence." (Daytona Beach News-Journal, October 29, 2012)

It is such socialization, along with the movement, that our instructor, Gabriela Trotta, tries to promote in her classes.

"It opened a whole new world to me," she said of her introduction to Dance for PD. (Daytona Beach News-Journal, Oct. 29, 2012)

Programs like Dance for PD or similar support groups can ease the feelings of isolation that Parkinson's can create.

This can be seen in the way Gabriela welcomes new members to her classes. She has each person perform a body movement and give their name. The rest of the class then follows suit, mimicking the movement and echoing the name.

Helga, a Parkinson's sufferer in her 80s, considers such interaction as a side benefit of staying active.

"The socialization is not why I joined Dance for PD, but it has become part of the reason for sticking with it," she said before a class. "Everything you do can be social if you want."

But not everyone is comfortable being open about their illness, especially in the beginning.

Chapter 13:
Uncomfortable with the Issue

Hialeah, Florida resident Marilyn Garateix didn't like to talk about her Parkinson's at first.

From her diagnosis in 2008 until 2015, when the former newspaper editor wrote an article about her battle with the chronic disorder for the Washington Post, Marilyn kept her illness hidden from everyone except for a select few.

It was a reprint of that article in the Tampa Bay Times that prompted me to contact Garateix and ask if we could talk.

Self-described as a very independent person who wants to maintain that freedom as long as possible, this single woman in her 50s told me she didn't want to deal with all the "questions and sympathetic stuff" that likely would arise if early news of her Parkinson's had come out.

"I was very uncomfortable with the issue becoming about me," Marilyn said while taking time away from a family trip to watch her nephew play in a youth baseball tournament in Kissimmee to talk with me. "As journalists, we are trained to focus on other people and focus on the story. I did not want to become the story."

Marilyn said her symptoms emerged in her 40s and the more she realized what the tremor in her thumb and the cramping of her left foot might represent, the less she wanted to discuss her problem.

At the time of her diagnosis, Marilyn was striving to earn an MBA, while working full-time as a journalist, and attempting to adopt a child. With all those distractions, she believed Parkinson's was something she could deal with eventually.

"Nobody knew I had Parkinson's. My tremor only came out when I was stressed," she said. "I kept the stress under control, so why bring all that down on me?"

She wasn't even sure she had the disorder at first, saying her neurologist spent months ruling everything else out before referring her to a Parkinson's disease specialist.

Marilyn quashed her own fears that she might have the disorder by telling herself that, as a Hispanic woman in her early 40s, she didn't fit the demographic profile of the typical

Parkinson's patient; elderly, white and male. This, despite her uncle having Parkinson's.

Describing her uncle as smart, funny and one of the most positive people in the world, Marilyn said Parkinson's was how she defined him growing up. It was how she knew him, and she didn't want the disease to similarly define her in the eyes of her own niece and nephew.

"I wanted to define Parkinson's," she said.

She said it took her a year to build up the courage to tell her parents, especially her father, of her illness because of her desire to remain independent.

"I wanted to cope with it first," she said. "I didn't want to be any less than I was before."

Additionally, Marilyn said it took her a long time to understand the disease.

"I am someone who has to know what is going on. I was very open about everything except this."

One of the biggest challenges Marilyn said she initially faced was how to manage her Parkinson's symptoms while, at the same time, managing her position as education editor of the Tampa Bay (Florida) Times newspaper.

"I wanted to keep it separate from my job," she said.

But that was not the only challenge she encountered. When it became evident her doctor couldn't tell her how bad her symptoms were going to get, Marilyn decided to give up her personal and professional dreams. Instead, she became hell-bent on meeting the disease head-on. She was determined to get the most out of life before the disorder took it from her.

The result of this was she became reckless, shopping like crazy, as well as drinking and partying heavily. While at the same time, she began ignoring such mundane tasks as paying her bills or taking care of her house.

Marilyn said she also embraced the four stages of grief: denial, anger, depression and bargaining. It was this attitude that eventually cost her both her house and her job. (Washington Post, 2015)

"I am a big planner. I plan everything out. I was going to get my MBA, adopt a child, become a managing editor, on and on," she said. "Parkinson's stopped all that. It all went out the window and I didn't know what to replace it with."

Marilyn said she finally hit rock bottom when she found herself lying in a fetal position on the bathroom floor of a bar while having a panic attack. That led to a trip to a hospital where an emergency room physician read her the riot act for drinking while taking prescription medications. It was at that moment, she realized if she kept her Parkinson's hidden any longer it was going to do her in.

"I needed to tell someone," Marilyn said. So, she let her bosses at the Times know of her diagnosis.

"They were great," she said.

Little by little, the circle of the informed grew. With one notable exception, the reporters on her team. Marilyn said she didn't inform them of the illness until she had decided to leave the newspaper to be closer to her parents in South Florida.

"I didn't want them to think I was leaving because of them," she explained. "Many people don't understand what it is like living with Parkinson's disease, and the newsrooms of this world are not the most supportive environments."

Marilyn admits she probably would have dealt with things differently if she had been diagnosed with an illness other than Parkinson's.

"I am very conscious of other people's perceptions (of me)," Marilyn said. "I was someone who did not slow down. Parkinson's slowed me down. I would multi-task aggressively; now I could not."

Using her passion for shoes to illustrate her point, she said Parkinson's may have taken many things from her, but she is determined not to let it win in the end.

"I am a shoe lover like you would not believe. I used to wear heels and now I can't (because of Parkinson's). I have to wear sneakers, but I am determined to wear fashionable sneakers," she said with a grin as she showed off her footwear.

Marilyn calls Parkinson's "an insidious sort of disease."

"When you have cancer, you have cancer and doctors can attack it," she said. "Then you either still have cancer or you don't. But with Parkinson's, you have to deal with one symptom after another. It is a degenerative disease. You can ask when it is going to end, but it doesn't end. I tell all my friends I know what it is like to be old already," said Marilyn.

Whatever Parkinson's disease took from Marilyn, it also provided her with the motivation to take on a very uncharacteristic challenge, something physical and visible. She decided to follow in her brother's (an Ironman triathlete) footsteps and run in a 5-kilometer road race before she turned 50 years old.

"I knew if I did something radically different with the Parkinson's, then I could do anything," she said.

And five days before her 50th birthday, Marilyn accomplished her goal, completing the almost 3.2-mile course in 51 minutes and 38 seconds. (Washington Post, 2015)

She credits her Parkinson's with spurring her on. According to Marilyn, the more she experienced a symptom while training for the race, the greater effort she put in.

"For me, it is about fighting," she said. "If I can get mad at Parkinson's, it helps me be able to deal with it."

In the seven years between diagnosis and crossing that finish line, Marilyn said her life was all about Parkinson's. But when this volunteer

CEO of a Miami-area non-profit organization and freelance writer completed her self-imposed challenge, she experienced a moment when the illness was no longer all-consuming. It was that awakening that prompted her to go public with her most personal battle, which, in the long run, helped her sort things out.

Marilyn still resents having Parkinson's, but she now focuses on living with it. And since everyone will eventually know she has the disorder, she believes she doesn't have to tell anyone anything until she absolutely wants to.

"Parkinson's is a challenge," Marilyn said. "It is something I have to battle, but at all times, I am the boss."

A Different Perspective

In 2013, Don Harris, an 80-year-old retired journalist from Palm Coast, Florida, had a specific motive for wanting to discuss his Parkinson's with anyone who would listen.

Don was hoping to develop a network of people as open as himself, who were willing to share their experiences with the disorder. Unfortunately, his efforts proved disappointing.

"It is discouraging that there are no support groups in Palm Coast," Don said while he waited for the annual Parkinson's Association of Greater Daytona Beach's "Sole Support" fun walk fundraiser to begin. This is no longer the case.

Support groups like the Daytona Beach association provide a forum where sufferers can exchange ideas about such topics as how to maintain a good quality of life. Creating interest in such a forum was the goal Don hoped to achieve with his fellow walkers.

The self-described pack-rat, who was diagnosed in 2003, said documents and research papers have their uses, but personal stories offer more insight, and since Parkinson's symptoms are as individual as its sufferers, he believes such connections are important.

"You can get information on the latest research from doctors, but you get a different type of information from the people who have Parkinson's," Don said. "There is more of an impact when you talk with other patients. You set up a bond."

Don's wife of more than 50 years, Frances, nodded in agreement while sitting next to her husband as she kept a protective eye on him.

"Sometimes I care for him and sometimes he cares for me," she quipped.

Frances said when the couple lived in Virginia, just outside Washington DC, they would attend Parkinson's disease support group meetings all the time. At these meetings, people would discuss all aspects of the disease, such as what drugs they were taking for their symptoms.

"This would work for that, but when others tried it, it would not work for them," she said. "Different medications work differently on different people."

The couple said they don't depend solely on support groups for their information, sometimes it comes from other sources like a book they recently read authored by a Young Onset Parkinson's patient, whose name they couldn't recall.

"He wrote about his different adventures," Frances said, "and he was very, very positive."

Not Advertising It

M.J. (no relation to the author and who asked his full name not be used), said once his Parkinson's was confirmed, he didn't try to conceal his condition, but he didn't advertise it either.

"When you have a tremor, a patient doesn't want to see you trying to give them an IV," the former radiological technician said while sitting in his beachside New Smyrna Beach home.

M.J. was diagnosed in 2002 at the age of 44. The first sign was a twitching finger.

"I thought I was nervous," he said.

It wasn't until later that he realized something was wrong.

M.J. and his wife, a nurse, were on a road trip to St. Augustine, Florida, when they came upon a traffic accident on Interstate 95. They stopped to assist the victims, but when the couple got back into their car, M.J. said the tremors in his legs were so severe he was unable to drive.

"I knew that was not normal," he said.

He went to see a doctor in hopes the tremors were something other than Parkinson's disease, but by the second doctor visit, he began to suspect the worst.

"I had worked with a lot of neurological patients," M.J. said of his career in the radiological department of a New Smyrna Beach hospital. He continued to work for about a decade after his diagnosis before deciding to retire.

"I was glad to get out when I did," he said. "I could not do the work as well, either physically or mentally, as I once did."

M.J. now receives Social Security disability insurance and spends most of his time at his computer or watching television.

"I am not really sure what to do (with myself)," he said.

M.J. is stiff and moves slowly as he lifts himself off the couch. He said tasks that once came easy are now difficult, and some he can't do at all. Although, he joked, "I can take a nap at almost any time."

M.J. is not the only member of his family with Parkinson's disease. He said a half-sister was diagnosed at age 67.

"It's almost as if you live long enough, you are going to get Parkinson's," he said.

Such tales may communicate the different ways a Parkinson's patient might isolate themselves from the world around them, but there are times when talking isn't enough to avoid this problem.

Chapter 14:
Ups and downs

Jerry Ingate tries to keep positive, especially when it comes to dealing with his Parkinson's. But when he forgets, his wife of five decades, Rosemarie, is quick to remind him.

"I tell him to snap out of it. I won't let him feel sorry for himself," she said as the couple sat down inside the Port Orange YMCA after an exercise class. "It is what it is, and you have to deal with it."

One way Jerry deals with his illness is with lots of exercise. When residing at their North Carolina home, Jerry said he works out with a group of cardiac patients three times a week at a local hospital.

"I am the only Parkinson's patient," he said. "They are a great group of people and a lot of fun. It is great being with all those people who are trying to strengthen their bodies."

The couple found a similar situation while visiting their winter residence in New Smyrna Beach when they joined the Dance for PD program at the local YMCA in 2016. Twice per week, Jerry and Rosemarie gathered with other Parkinson's sufferers and their caregivers for an hour-long session of exercise and socialization.

Rosemarie initially had some trepidation about how her husband would react to his fellow classmates, particularly if their symptoms were worse than his own.

"I hoped it would not be too terribly depressing," she said. "I thought it might put him into a funk."

The exact opposite proved true.

"I enjoy the classes tremendously," Jerry said.

Unfortunately, when the couple traveled south during the winter of 2017, Jerry's situation wasn't as positive. His already rail-thin frame was even thinner, and his tremor had encompassed his entire upper torso.

"He is having a rough time," Rosemarie said. "There are some good days and some not so good days."

She speculated this downward turn may be caused by a new infusion drug treatment Jerry was using. The system is supposed to route dopamine around the digestive system, thus getting it to his brain quicker and reducing its "off times" when the medication is least effective. However, the results aren't always consistent for Jerry.

He said the biggest physical impact of his Parkinson's has been a loss of mobility, strength and stamina, mainly on his right side. When his drug therapy does what it's supposed to, he said he is able to function, but when it doesn't work, the disease leaves him almost incapable of movement.

Although he feels more upbeat and stronger after exercising, Jerry said his routine needs to be more than once or twice a week to be effective.

"It's a longevity thing," he said.

Looking back on his history with Parkinson's, this former financial advisor for Morgan-Stanley said he began to display symptoms while on a Russian vacation with Rosemarie in 2008.

The couple were on their way home, via a cruise to Holland, when a doctor aboard the ship told Jerry he should have himself checked out because he might have Parkinson's disease.

"I was shaking a bit on the boat," Jerry said.

There were earlier hints too, such as the loss of his senses of smell and taste about a year prior to the trip, he said. "That should have been a tip off."

Rosemarie said she suspected something was wrong even earlier, but Jerry didn't put much credence in her suspicions; that is until they were confirmed by an Asheville, NC, neurology group.

"He would not listen to me," she lamented.

Jerry's physical well-being is not the only casualty of Parkinson's, it has also altered the couple's relationship.

"I'm more protective of him," Rosemarie said. "I am his advocate."

And she said she is not alone in treating her husband differently as a result of his illness.

"Sophisticated people see it right away," Rosemarie said of the Parkinson's tremors that are evident in Jerry's extremities. And because of this, she speculates people are more accommodating toward him.

"Although that could be our age," she mused.

Using a recent trip to Turkey as an example, she spoke of a young man who not only assisted the couple with their carry-on bags as they boarded the aircraft, but offered to help them at flight's end, too. In another case, the couple said, their tour guide noticed Jerry was having a problem negotiating the step up into the minivan they were using. He mentioned this to a friend who quickly fashioned a wooden step-stool for Jerry's use.

"That makes me encouraged about human beings," Rosemarie said.

She added that day-to-day activities also take more planning because of her husband's Parkinson's.

Using Jerry's fondness for soup to illustrate the point, Rosemarie said, "soup can be very hard to eat (for a person with Parkinson's) when you are out (at a restaurant)." Instead of a bowl, the couple asks for Jerry's soup to be served in a mug. That way, he can grasp the handle and sip it rather than having to use a spoon.

At first, Jerry admitted he had some concerns about what people might say about him seeking such accommodations, but his wife had no such thoughts.

"Who cares? If you take it in stride, people will take it in stride." said Rosemarie. "And if someone says something, then they are no friend of yours."

Jerry says if he could travel back in time and give his younger self some advice about what to do in the future with Parkinson's disease, he would tell himself, "keep a positive mental attitude and get some exercise."

Given the same opportunity, Rosemarie said she would encourage Parkinson's patients and their caregivers not to postpone things that are important to them—like trips.

"And remember things could always be worse."

Chapter 15:
A Final Thought

By sharing their stories, the Parkinson's community establishes a bedrock from which we can all continue our fight against the disease. And while it is a battle we must believe one day that we will win, we cannot hang our hats on hope alone. Until that day, my fellow "movers and shakers" must strive to squeeze everything possible from each opportunity that presents itself. By doing so, we can look back upon our lives without regret.

Acknowledgements

First, and most importantly, I want to thank the dozens of my fellow Parkies who allowed me to interview them. They put up with my seemingly endless stream of personal, and at times intrusive, questions that I needed to get answered so I could accumulate the facts and stories that make up this book. Without their patience and that of their caregivers, these pages would have never been possible. My eternal gratitude to you all.

I would like to thank my father for his support, suggestions and encouragement while I was writing this book. Without his assistance, it might never have become a reality.

In addition, I want to give a shout out to my friends who read my preliminary manuscripts and gave their invaluable input as to what to include in and exclude from this final version. Most especially, to Laura Williams who gave her time to provide an early edit that helped me put my thoughts into a coherent order.

Thank you all

About the Author

Mark I. Johnson spent 30 years as a newspaper photographer and reporter before his career was cut short when he was diagnosed at the age of 45 with Young-Onset Parkinson's disease in November 2006. Although he worked for another seven years after his diagnosis, fatigue, tremors and other Parkinson's symptoms eventually lead Johnson to retire early from the profession that he loved.

After his retirement, Johnson decided to put the skills he learned as a reporter to use by writing a book that outlined the experiences he and other Parkinson's sufferers have undergone while battling this chronic degenerative disease.

Johnson is 57 years old and lives in Edgewater, Florida with his wife Beverly. Much of his time is taken up by his continuing effort to stay in motion through his attendance in various exercise programs. When he isn't working to keep his Parkinson's at bay, he enjoys photography and saltwater fly fishing.

Fellow Parkies

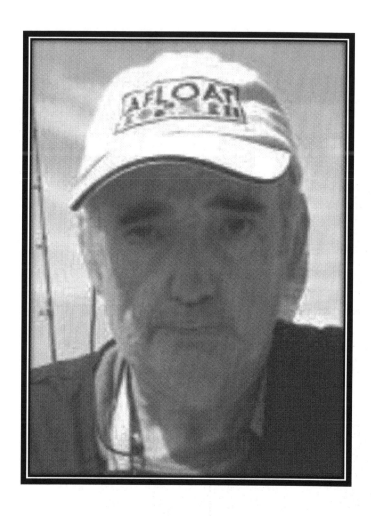

Roger David Borrow

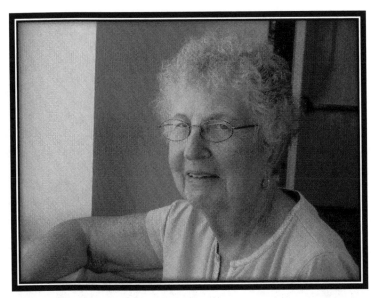

Helga

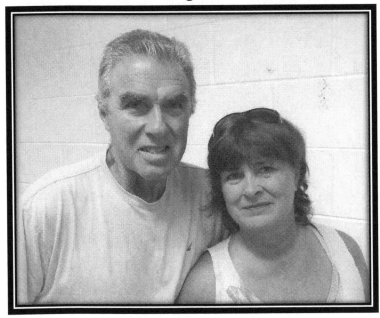

John and Pat Mirabella

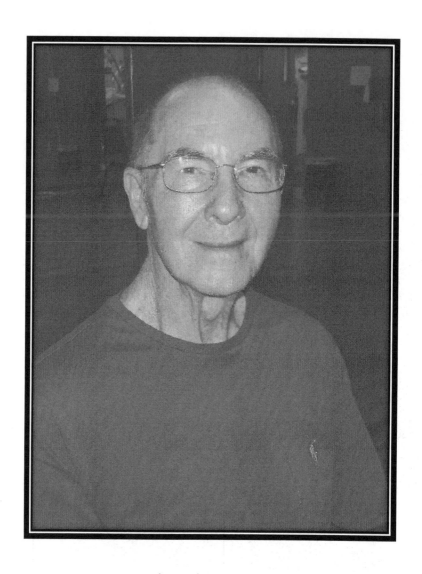

Jerry Ingate

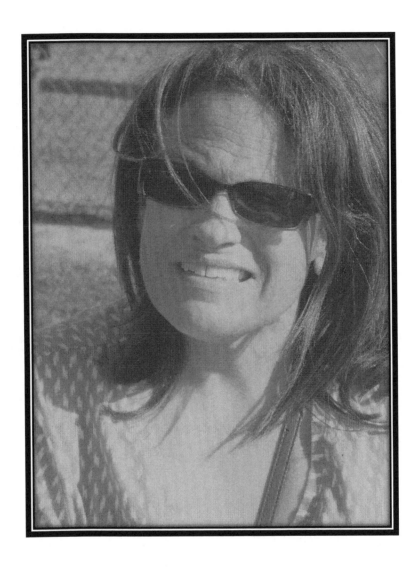

Marilyn Garateix

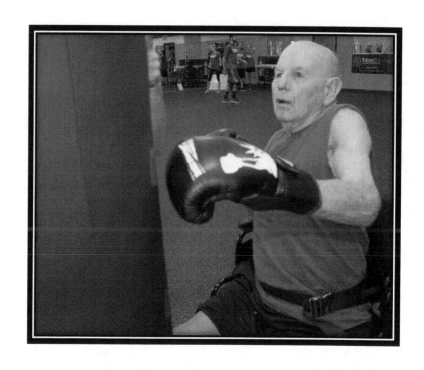

Maynard Kern

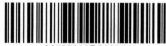

Made in the USA
Columbia, SC
27 November 2018